CHAIR YOGA REVOLUTION FOR SENIORS

A Therapeutic Approach to Daily Exercises to Improve Strength, Increase Endurance, and Enhance Balance to Promote Mobility

Shelley Carroll, MPT

Copyright © Shelley Carroll, MPT. 2025 - All rights reserved.

The content contained within this book may not be reproduced, duplicated, or transmitted without direct written permission from the author or the publisher.

Under no circumstances will any blame or legal responsibility be held against the publisher or author for any damages, reparation, or monetary loss due to the information contained within this book. Either directly or indirectly. You are responsible for your own choices, actions, and the resulting consequences.

Legal Notice:

This book is copyright-protected. This book is intended for personal use only. You cannot amend, distribute, sell, use, quote, or paraphrase any part of the content within this book without the consent of the author or publisher.

Disclaimer Notice:

Please note that the information contained within this document is for educational and entertainment purposes only. All efforts have been made to present accurate, up-to-date, and reliable information, complete and accurate. No warranties of any kind are declared or implied. Readers acknowledge that the author is not engaging in the rendering of legal, financial, medical, or professional advice. The author and publisher are not responsible for any adverse effects from using the information contained herein. Always consult a healthcare professional for your individual health needs. The content within this book has been derived from various sources. Please consult a licensed professional before attempting any techniques outlined in this book.

By reading this document, the reader agrees that under no circumstances is the author responsible for any losses, direct or indirect, which are incurred as a result of the use of the information contained within this document, including, but not limited to, errors, omissions, or inaccuracies.

Shelley Carrol MPT

Table of Contents

Copyright © Shelley Carroll, MPT. 2025 - All rights reserved. 2

PREFACE 5

INTRODUCTION 6

CHAPTER 1: FOUNDATIONS OF CHAIR YOGA FOR SENIORS 9
   1.1 Understanding Chair Yoga: Benefits for Seniors 9
   1.2 Creating a Safe Exercise Environment at Home 11
   1.3 Mitigating Falls in the Home 12
   1.4 Essential Chair Yoga Equipment 13
   1.5 Breathing Techniques for Improved Function and Relaxation 14
   1.6 The Mind-Body Connection 16

CHAPTER 2: CHAIR YOGA AND COMMON HEALTH CHALLENGES 18
   2.1 Managing Arthritis Pain with Gentle Movements 18
   Interactive Element: 19
   2.2 Exercises to Support Bone Health 23
   Interactive Element: 24
   2.3 Improving Cardiovascular Health with Chair Yoga 27
   Interactive Element: 27
   2.4 Managing and Maintaining Weight with Chair Exercises 29
   2.5 Connecting Exercise with Improved Mental Health 30

CHAPTER 3: NUTRITION AND HYDRATION FOR OPTIMAL PERFORMANCE 33
   3.1 Protein Power: Building Muscles and Tissues 33
   3.2 Hydration Essentials: Preventing Dehydration 35
   3.3 Nutritional Tips for Enhanced Energy Levels 37
   3.4 Nutritional Tips for Post-Exercise Recovery 38

CHAPTER 4: BUILDING STRENGTH THROUGH CHAIR EXERCISES 41
   4.1 Upper Body Strengthening 41
   Interactive Element: Upper Body Exercises 42
   4.2 Lower Body Strengthening 48
   Interactive Element: Lower Body Exercises 48
   4.3 Core Strength Exercises for Improved Balance 54
   Interactive Element: Core Exercises 55

CHAPTER 5: ENHANCING BALANCE THROUGH EXERCISE 62
   5.1 Balance and Fall Prevention Techniques 63
   Interactive Element: Balance Exercises 64

CHAPTER 6: CARDIOVASCULAR FOCUS 76
   6.1 Using a Chair for Cardiovascular Exercise 76
   Personal Reflection: Setting Your Heart Health Goals 77
   Interactive Element: Cardiovascular Exercises 78

CHAPTER 7: ADAPTING CHAIR YOGA FOR LIMITED MOBILITY 82
7.1 Using Support for Safe Standing Exercises 83

CHAPTER 8 USING PROGRESS LOGS FOR MOTIVATION 84
8.1 The Benefits of Tracking Progress 84
8.2 Establish a Realistic Timeline for Improvement 85
SAMPLE ROUTINES TO CONSIDER 87

CHAPTER 9: GENTLE STRETCHING FOR JOINT, MUSCLE, AND MENTAL HEALTH 92
9.1 Holistic Benefits of Stretching 92
9.2 Range of Motion for Improved Mobility and Safety 94
Interactive Element: Stretching Checklist 95
9.3 Reduce Stiffness Throughout the Day 102

CHAPTER 10: CREATING A SUSTAINABLE EXERCISE HABIT 103
10.1 Overcoming Common Exercise Barriers 104
10.2 Setting Achievable Fitness Goals 106
10.3 Keeping Motivation High with Diverse Routines 108
10.4 Overcoming Exercise Plateaus 109

CHAPTER 11: PROMOTING RELAXATION AND STRESS RELIEF 111
11.1 Relaxation Techniques 111
11.2 Add Relaxation into Daily Routines 113
11.3 Mindfulness Practices for Seniors 114

CHAPTER 12: INSPIRING OTHERS: SHARING YOUR JOURNEY 116

Conclusion 118

References 120

Preface

In my over 10 years working with the senior population, I have seen an increasing number of patients diagnosed with complications related to dehydration and protein-calorie malnutrition. While this book offers guided exercises to help improve mobility and strength, I felt adding a section regarding diet, nutrition, and hydration was very important.

Please consult your physician before starting any new exercise program, modifying your diet, or taking supplements. Requesting lab tests to check your body chemistry is a wise step to determine whether you have deficiencies in nutrients, proteins, vitamins, or minerals.

This book is based on my experience as a physical therapist and is intended for informational and educational purposes only. It is not designed to offer medical advice, diagnosis, or treatment.

Before starting any exercise program, making dietary changes, or altering your health regimen, please consult your physician or a qualified healthcare provider.

Introduction

Imagine waking up with confidence, moving through your day efficiently, and engaging in activities you once thought were beyond your reach. This isn't merely a dream; it's a reality that chair yoga can make possible. Every session enhances your physical strength, balance, and flexibility. Embark on a journey that promises to transform your daily routine and elevate the quality and vibrancy of your life.

As you turn these pages, you'll dive into the multifaceted benefits of this practice, designed with your unique needs in mind. Chair yoga goes beyond physical health, aiming to reclaim your independence, reduce pain, and foster an invigorating sense of well-being. By integrating simple, structured exercises into your daily life, you'll navigate everyday tasks with newfound confidence and a sense of a fresh start each day.

This book isn't just a guide; it's your companion in creating a safe, nurturing exercise environment at home using everyday items. You'll learn how to connect endurance and strength with nutrition and hydration, crafting a holistic approach to wellness. Each chapter offers practical advice, ranging from soothing breathing techniques to advanced poses, along with suggestions for adapting them to varying levels of mobility.

With 27 years of experience as a physical therapist, including over a decade dedicated to geriatric home health care, I've amassed a wealth of knowledge. I've guided countless seniors through recovery from hospitalizations, illnesses, surgeries, and falls. My work involves crafting tailored home exercise programs for individuals with diverse mobility and strength levels, providing me with a profound insight into the unique challenges of aging and the best practices for successful rehabilitation.

I recall a spirited woman in her late seventies, newly recovered from hip surgery following a fall. Initially hesitant due to pain, she embraced chair exercises with my encouragement. Her journey from simple seated exercises to standing ones was remarkable. Her strength, balance, and confidence soared, lighting up her life with newfound independence. This, among countless other stories, inspired me to write "Chair Yoga Revolution for Seniors," a book designed to empower you through simple, effective routines that utilize everyday household items to enhance your strength, endurance, and balance.

Chair yoga offers unique benefits for seniors. It safely enhances physical health by improving flexibility, strength, and balance while boosting mental well-being, reducing stress, and promoting better sleep. Studies support the notion that regular exercise can improve mood and cognitive function, making chair yoga a vital component of a healthy lifestyle.

You might be concerned about starting an exercise routine, doubt your fitness level, or think yoga is only for the young and flexible. Let me reassure you that chair yoga is accessible to everyone. The exercises here are safe, adaptable, and designed for all mobility levels, allowing you to practice at your own pace with modifications to match your needs.

This book stands out because of its practical approach. By utilizing items like water bottles and grocery bags for resistance exercises, fitness becomes inexpensive and accessible. It also includes targeted nutritional advice, emphasizing the role of protein in muscle health and the importance of hydration. This comprehensive strategy equips you with tools for optimal physical wellness.

Engaging with "Chair Yoga Revolution for Seniors" will help unlock vitality and allow you to embrace a more fulfilling life. Thank you for trusting me to guide you through this empowering adventure. Let's make every day an opportunity for growth and enjoyment.

Chapter 1: Foundations of Chair Yoga for Seniors

Once, I worked with a gentleman whose determination and resilience left a lasting impression on me. He suffered a stroke that significantly impacted his mobility, leaving him dependent on others for basic tasks. He was hesitant about exercising, fearing he would fall. Yet, when introduced to chair yoga, he discovered a practice that accommodated his physical limitations and fostered gradual progress. Using a simple chair, he began with gentle stretches and movements. Over time, his sitting balance returned, his strength improved, and his confidence skyrocketed. This chapter begins your exploration into chair yoga, a practice that, like for this gentleman, can offer profound benefits regardless of your current physical condition.

1.1 Understanding Chair Yoga: Benefits for Seniors

Chair yoga accommodates a wide range of physical abilities, making it an inclusive fitness option. Unlike more traditional yoga forms, chair yoga employs the support of a chair, allowing you to execute poses safely and confidently. This makes it particularly beneficial for individuals with limited mobility and at risk of falling, as it provides a foundation of support that can be adjusted according to your needs. The adaptability of chair yoga means you can tailor exercises to suit your level, ensuring that you engage in safe and effective movements. It provides a perfect entry point into exercise, especially for those apprehensive about more strenuous routines. Chair yoga is for everyone, regardless of your current physical condition.

The benefits of chair yoga are multifaceted, encompassing physical and mental improvements. Physically, you can expect enhanced flexibility and joint health, as the gentle movements help to lubricate and strengthen the joints. Improved flexibility can lead to decreased stiffness and pain, which are common issues that many people face as they age. Additionally, weight management becomes more attainable as your mobility improves, which in turn contributes to overall health and vitality.

Furthermore, chair exercises significantly enhance core strength, thereby reducing the risk of falls, a critical concern for seniors.

Mentally, the practice encourages relaxation and stress reduction, promoting clarity and a sense of calm.

Supporting these claims, a study published in the Journal of Geriatric Health highlights the effectiveness of chair yoga in improving functional fitness and daily life activities among older adults. The research involved participants who, after 12 weeks of chair yoga therapy, showed marked improvements in muscle strength, balance, and agility. These findings underscore the role of chair yoga as a credible and effective fitness regimen for seniors. Professionals in the geriatric health field also endorse chair yoga, emphasizing its ability to enhance the quality of life while accommodating the unique challenges older adults face.

Common misconceptions about yoga and exercise often deter seniors from participating. Some may believe that exercises pose a danger, particularly for those with existing health concerns. However, with proper guidance, chair yoga can reduce the risk of falls, improve mobility, and support cardiovascular health. Another misconception is that age is a barrier to starting an exercise routine. In truth, regular physical activity enhances muscle strength, flexibility, mood, and cognitive function, proving beneficial regardless of when you begin. Many also believe that only cardiovascular exercises are valuable, yet strength and flexibility exercises are equally vital in maintaining muscle mass and bone density, preventing injuries, and supporting daily activities. The notion that exercise is ineffective for chronic conditions is another falsehood. With proper supervision, exercise can help alleviate symptoms of conditions such as arthritis and heart disease, thereby improving function and quality of life.

Chair yoga offers a transformative approach to exercise, designed with your needs in mind. Whether you're new to exercise or seeking a gentle yet effective routine, chair yoga offers a path to improved mobility and a more active lifestyle. Seated exercises offer a remarkable advantage for individuals with mobility challenges, providing a gateway to physical activity without the risk of overstraining or compromising safety.

1.2 Creating a Safe Exercise Environment at Home

Establishing a safe and adequate space for chair yoga within your home is the first step toward a rewarding practice. The environment you choose should not only accommodate your physical needs but also provide a sense of comfort and motivation. Start by selecting an area that offers ample room to move freely without obstruction. Non-slip mats or rugs prevent slips and falls, ensuring that each movement is executed with confidence. Adequate lighting is crucial; it enhances visibility and contributes to a brighter, more inviting atmosphere. An organized, well-lit space can transform your home into a sanctuary for personal wellness.

One cannot overemphasize the importance of safety when engaging in any exercise. The area you designate for your practice should remain clear of obstacles. Remove any clutter or loose items that could pose a tripping hazard. Choose a solid chair with a sturdy frame and in good condition, with a firm seat and no wheels. A chair that wobbles or feels unstable can undermine your confidence and increase the risk of injury. The seat should be firm, providing a stable base that supports your weight without sagging. Armrests can offer additional support, aiding balance and providing a point of leverage. If the chair has adjustable armrests, position them so that you can rest your arms comfortably, without straining your shoulders. Check the chair's height in relation to your body to ensure your feet can rest flat on the floor when seated. This helps maintain good posture and alignment, making it easier to move between sitting and standing, thus reducing strain and enhancing ease of movement.

A space dedicated to chair yoga should feel inviting and reflect your unique style. Incorporating elements that resonate with you can enhance your connection to the practice, making it a regular part of your routine. Consider the room's color scheme and how it affects your mood. Soft, calming colors may promote relaxation, while brighter hues can energize and invigorate. Music can also play a role in setting the tone for your practice. Choose soothing melodies or nature sounds to accompany your sessions, creating an auditory backdrop that complements your movements.

1.3 Mitigating Falls in the Home

Creating a safer home environment is crucial for reducing the risk of falls, a concern that often weighs on the minds of seniors and their families. The first step in minimizing fall hazards is to assess your living space with a critical eye, identifying potential risks that could lead to an accident.

Loose rugs, for instance, are common culprits for slips and falls. Secure them with non-slip backing or remove them entirely to ensure a stable walking surface. Clutter and electrical cords pose a threat, obstructing pathways and increasing the risk of tripping. Keeping pathways clear of furniture and other obstacles further enhances safety, providing a direct route free from hindrances that could cause an accident.

Another effective modification involves installing grab bars in strategic areas such as bathrooms and staircases. These bars provide sturdy support, enabling you to maintain balance when navigating potentially slippery surfaces or transitioning between different levels of your home. They offer peace of mind, particularly in spaces where falls are more likely, such as the bathroom, where water and smooth surfaces can create a hazardous situation.

It is paramount to ensure that your home is well-lit. Nightlights in hallways and bathrooms can guide you during nocturnal trips, reducing the likelihood of disorientation or missteps in the dark. Proper lighting in staircases and entryways is also essential, allowing you to see clearly and navigate safely.

Mindfulness plays a significant role in fall prevention by enhancing awareness and focus during movement. Mindful walking involves paying close attention to each step, consciously feeling the ground beneath your feet, and maintaining an even pace. This focus reduces distractions and encourages intentional movement, minimizing the risk of missteps.

For seniors, wearing the proper attire also plays a significant role in fall prevention. Good-fitting footwear provides necessary support and stability, reducing the risk of tripping. Non-slip socks are essential for indoor safety, providing a secure grip on various surfaces to prevent slips. Properly fitting pants ensure freedom of movement without the risk of getting caught on the ground.

Assessing and modifying your living space, integrating mindfulness with movement, and wearing properly fitting attire all contribute to a safer and more independent lifestyle. This combination forms a robust strategy for reducing the risk of falls, empowering you to live more securely and independently.

1.4 Essential Chair Yoga Equipment

In preparing for chair yoga, actively search your home for practical exercise tools. You'll find a treasure trove of potential equipment ready for repurposing. Take water bottles, for instance. When filled to your desired weight, they transform into excellent hand weights, ideal for arm exercises and strength-building routines. They provide the resistance needed to tone muscles without the cost or bulk of traditional dumbbells. Their familiar shape and weight make them comfortable to handle, reducing any intimidation you might feel when beginning a new exercise.

Consider the humble, sturdy bag, a standard item with uncommon potential. By adding weight, you create a customizable tool for resistance training, allowing you to adjust the challenge to match your strength and progress. The adaptability of bags filled with household items ensures a versatile training aid accommodating varying degrees of difficulty and fitness levels.

Towels can often be indispensable for stretching exercises. They serve as extensions of your limbs, aiding in reaching those muscles requiring extra attention. By looping a towel around your foot or hand, you can increase the range and depth of a stretch, enhancing flexibility without straining. This simple tool can help maintain alignment and support, which is crucial for safe and effective stretching, especially for those with limited flexibility.

Large, sturdy books can serve as effective yoga blocks, providing support and stability during poses that require balance and extended reach. These makeshift blocks can help you maintain proper form, reducing the risk of injury while you build confidence and strength. Their solid structure offers the support needed for various poses, allowing you to deepen your practice and gradually improve your flexibility.

Using familiar household items simplifies the transition into chair yoga, making it less intimidating and more engaging. These everyday objects bring comfort to your practice, reducing anxiety and the need for specialized equipment, thus encouraging regular participation.

When incorporating these items into your chair exercise practice, ensuring their safety and durability is paramount. Always check the integrity of your equipment before use. Ensure water bottles are securely closed to prevent spillage, and inspect bags for weak seams. Towels should be free from tears, and books should be sturdy enough to bear weight without collapsing. This attention to detail will safeguard your sessions, allowing you to focus on the benefits of your practice.

Also, you can purchase dumbbells, wrist or ankle weights, and elastic bands if you prefer them and can afford them. Local sports and fitness stores often carry a range of weights and resistance bands, allowing you to select items that match your current fitness level and will enable you to increase resistance as you gradually gain strength. Additionally, online retailers, such as specialized fitness websites, offer a wide selection with the convenience of home delivery.

I encourage you to embrace creativity in your exercise setups. Each home is unique; the best solutions often arise from personal ingenuity. Consider your space and resources, and tailor your setup to meet your specific needs. Whether rearranging furniture to create more room or experimenting with different household items, your imagination is your only limit. This flexibility in approach ensures that chair yoga is both effective and a personalized, fulfilling experience.

1.5 Breathing Techniques for Improved Function and Relaxation

When exercising, the breath is not merely a passive element but actively directs and enhances every movement, playing a pivotal role in the practice. Proper breathing fuels your body and mind, enhancing the fluidity and grace of each motion. By synchronizing breath with movement, you cultivate a rhythm that supports mindfulness, allowing you to remain present and focused. This harmonious integration of breath and movement transforms each pose into a meditation in motion, where the mind, body, and breath work in unison. Attentive breathing enhances concentration and clarity throughout your practice.

Breathing is not just about inhaling and exhaling during chair exercises; it's a tool that significantly enhances physical movements and focus. One of the most effective techniques is diaphragmatic breathing. This method engages the diaphragm, the muscle separating the chest from the abdomen, encouraging deeper and more efficient breaths.

- Begin by sitting comfortably, placing one hand on your chest and the other on your abdomen.
- Inhale deeply through the nose, allowing the diaphragm to drop and the rib cage and abdomen to expand.
- The hand on your belly should rise more than the one on your chest.
- Exhale slowly through pursed lips, feeling your abdomen contract.
- This breathing exercise improves lung capacity and fosters relaxation, which helps reduce stress

Alternate nostril breathing, another beneficial technique, promotes balance and clarity. It involves inhaling through one nostril while closing the other, then exhaling through the same nostril. To practice this technique, do the following:

- Sit upright, gently close the right nostril with your thumb, and inhale deeply through the left.
- Close the left nostril with your ring finger, release the right nostril, and exhale fully through the right.
- Continue this pattern, alternating nostrils with each breath.
- This technique, rooted in ancient yoga practices, enhances mental focus and stability and fosters calm alertness.

To illustrate these techniques further, imagine a typical exercise session: Gently lift your arms to shoulder height with each inhale, feeling your chest expand and your spine lengthen. Then, as you exhale, lower your arms, allowing your shoulders to relax, and press your feet firmly into the ground. This intentional pairing of breath with movement amplifies the exercise's physical benefits and deepens your engagement with the practice, cultivating a sense of inner peace and stability.

The benefits of these breathing techniques extend beyond the chair yoga session. Regular practice can lead to tangible health benefits, including increased lung capacity and improved respiratory efficiency. Focusing on deep, controlled breathing trains the lungs to take in more oxygen, enhancing endurance and stamina. Furthermore, these exercises may significantly reduce stress and anxiety levels.

Scientific studies support the effectiveness of breathing exercises in promoting health and well-being. For instance, research documented by the American Lung Association highlights how practices like diaphragmatic breathing can improve lung function and overall respiratory health. By cultivating these techniques, you can enhance your chair yoga practice and contribute to your long-term physical and mental health.

1.6 The Mind-Body Connection

The connection between the mind and body is a fundamental pillar. This practice promotes an understanding of how mental and physical health are intricately intertwined. As you engage in movements, each pose becomes an opportunity to cultivate mindfulness, allowing you to tune into the present moment and observe the sensations within your body. This awareness transforms a simple exercise into a holistic experience, where the mind is as much a part of the workout as the muscles themselves. By aligning movements with conscious thought, chair yoga encourages a deeper understanding of self, promoting mental clarity and physical well-being.

Mindful movement cultivates a state of mental calmness, helping to reduce the chaos of racing thoughts. Physical exercise acts as a bridge to mental clarity, providing a space to escape the stresses of daily life. As you move through poses, your mind becomes more centered, allowing you to experience a sense of peace and relaxation. This mental clarity is refreshing and essential for maintaining a balanced, healthy life.

The psychological benefits of regular exercise and chair yoga are profound. Engaging in these practices can reduce depression symptoms, as the release of endorphins and other neurotransmitters fosters a positive mood. Furthermore, regular practice enhances memory and concentration as the mind becomes accustomed to the discipline of focus and relaxation. This improvement in cognitive function can lead to a more alert and vibrant mind, enabling individuals to support daily activities and mental tasks with greater ease.

Consider setting intentions before starting your yoga practice to maintain a mindful approach throughout your session. These intentions can be simple, such as focusing on relaxation or embracing a positive mindset. By setting an intention, you guide your attention and enhance the quality of the exercises.

By embracing the mind-body connection through chair yoga, you are not merely engaging in physical exercise. This chapter invites you to explore these connections, encouraging a holistic approach to health that nurtures both the physical and the mental. Through mindful movement, relaxation, and reflection, you can achieve a more balanced and fulfilling life.

Chapter 2: Chair Yoga and Common Health Challenges

Chair yoga is a transformative, adaptable exercise modality perfect for seniors facing various health conditions commonly associated with aging. One of its paramount advantages is enhancing flexibility and joint mobility. This is particularly crucial for older adults, as it can substantially alleviate stiffness and reduce the discomfort associated with prevalent conditions such as arthritis.

Moreover, balance and strength emerge as critical focus areas, especially considering their direct correlation with an increased risk of falls among older adults. Chair yoga thoughtfully incorporates a variety of poses that gently yet effectively strengthen muscles and bolster stability, thereby markedly reducing the likelihood of falls. This aspect of chair yoga is indispensable in promoting a sense of physical confidence and autonomy among seniors.

In addition, chair yoga substantially improves circulation, a common concern for seniors, particularly those with conditions such as peripheral artery disease. Many chair yoga movements specifically involve leg exercises, which can significantly enhance blood flow and circulation, thus addressing such conditions with gentle, targeted activity.

Chair yoga, too, benefits mental wellness immensely. This form of exercise is a powerful tool for stress relief, anxiety reduction, and depression mitigation. Through meditative practices and focused breathing exercises, seniors can cultivate a serene state of mind, thereby enhancing their overall mental well-being.

In essence, chair yoga offers a comprehensive, accessible, and practical approach to senior health care. It embodies a holistic approach to maintaining or enhancing health and well-being, making it a valuable addition to a senior's daily routine.

2.1 Managing Arthritis Pain with Gentle Movements

For those battling arthritis, chair yoga has emerged as a promising ally in managing the often debilitating pain associated with this condition. Arthritis, characterized by inflammation and stiffness in the joints, usually restricts movement and diminishes quality of life. Yet, with its gentle and deliberate movements, exercise is particularly effective in enhancing the movement of the existing synovial fluid. This fluid acts as a cushion between bones, reducing friction and alleviating the persistent pain that arthritis can cause. Thus, through the gentle art of chair yoga, individuals with arthritis can find relief from pain and improve mobility.

Chair range-of-motion exercises are excellent for managing arthritis because they help maintain joint flexibility, reduce stiffness, and improve circulation without putting excessive strain on the body. When practiced daily or several times a week, these exercises can improve joint function and significantly reduce pain levels, supporting a more active and comfortable lifestyle, as various studies on yoga for arthritis management have shown.

Interactive Element:

Here are some of the best chair range-of-motion exercises tailored for arthritis. They focus on commonly affected areas such as the shoulders, wrists, hips, knees, and ankles.

SHOULDER ROLLS:

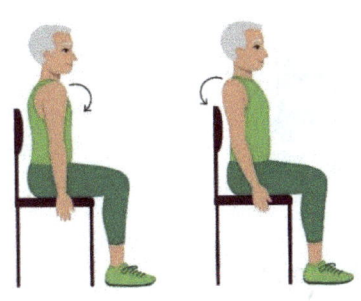

- Sit upright in a chair with arms relaxed at your sides.
- Slowly roll your shoulders forward in a circular motion for 10–15 seconds (5–10 rolls).
- Reverse direction and roll backward for another 10–15 seconds. Repeat 2–3 times.
- Keep movements smooth and avoid hunching.

Chair Yoga Revolution for Seniors

SEATED WRIST CIRCLES:

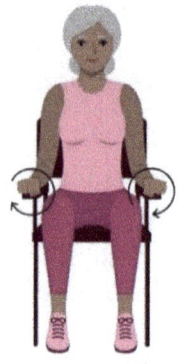

- Sit upright in a chair with forearms resting on your thighs or chair arms, with your wrists and hands extended past your knees or the end of the chair arms.
- Rotate wrists clockwise for 10–15 seconds, then counterclockwise.
- Perform 2–3 sets per direction.
- Start with small circles and increase their size if you feel comfortable.

SEATED MARCHING:

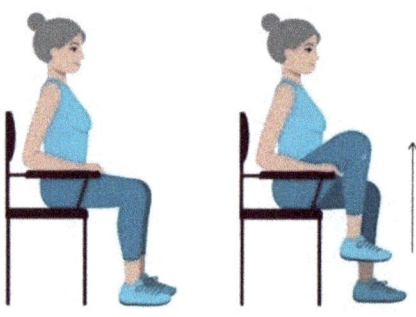

- Sit upright in a chair with your feet flat on the floor.
- Lift your right knee towards your chest as high as comfortably.
- Gently lower your leg back to the starting position.
- Repeat the motion with the other leg and alternate legs, doing 5-10 lifts per leg. Repeat 2–3 sets.
- Move slowly to avoid jarring the joints.

ANKLE CIRCLES:

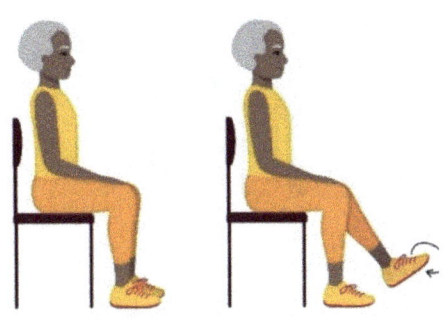

- Sit upright in a chair with your feet flat on the floor.
- Lift one foot slightly off the ground.
- Rotate your ankle clockwise for 10–15 seconds, then counterclockwise.
- Switch to the other ankle, and repeat 2–3 times per side.
- Point and flex toes during circles for added benefit.

SEATED KICKS:

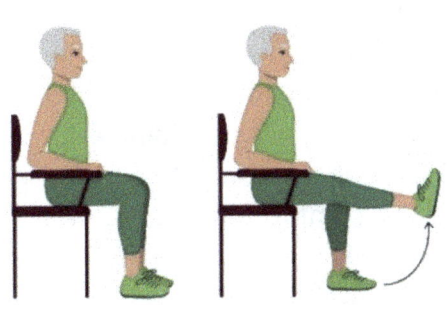

- Sit upright in a chair with your feet flat on the floor.
- Slowly extend one knee until it's straight (or as far as comfortable).
- Hold the extended position for 1-2 seconds, then slowly lower the leg back down.
- Alternate legs, doing 5-10 kicks per leg, and repeat 2–3 sets.

NECK ROLLS:

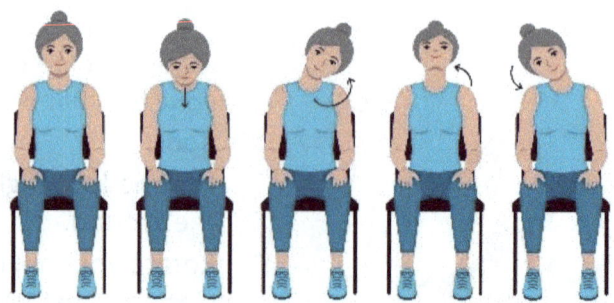

- Sit upright in a chair with your feet flat on the floor.
- Gently drop your chin to your chest and roll your head to the right in a circular motion, moving your ear toward your shoulder.
- Tilt your head back, then roll your head to the left in a circular motion, moving your ear toward your shoulder.
- Complete the circle by bringing your chin back to your chest.
- Do 5–10 circles clockwise, then reverse direction.
- Stop if you feel dizzy or discomfort.

As you begin to incorporate these exercises, it is crucial to prioritize safety and listen to your body's signals. The key to effective arthritis management through yoga lies in the execution of movements that are slow and mindful. This approach prevents overexertion and ensures you remain attuned to your body's needs, avoiding exercises that might trigger flare-ups. Over-stretching can exacerbate pain, so it is essential to move within limits that feel comfortable and sustainable. By maintaining a gentle pace and focusing on the quality of each movement, you create an environment where healing and relief can flourish

Alongside these movements, complementary lifestyle modifications can significantly bolster your arthritis management strategy. Heat therapy, for instance, is an excellent method for soothing sore joints. Applying a warm compress or soaking in a warm bath can relax muscles and improve circulation, providing immediate comfort. Additionally, dietary adjustments aimed at reducing inflammation can further enhance the benefits of your yoga practice.

Incorporating foods rich in omega-3 fatty acids, such as fish and flaxseeds, can help combat inflammation, while reducing intake of processed foods may decrease symptoms. Lastly, maintaining adequate hydration is crucial, as water is vital in keeping joints lubricated and functioning optimally. By ensuring your body is well-hydrated, you support the overall health of your joints, facilitating smoother movements and reducing friction.

Combined with consistent chair yoga practice, strategies like dietary adjustments or heat therapy create a comprehensive approach to managing arthritis pain. By embracing gentle movements and lifestyle changes, you can significantly improve joint function and reduce pain levels. This holistic approach empowers you to take control of your arthritis management, enhancing your quality of life and enabling you to engage in activities you enjoy. Begin exploring these strategies today to reclaim your mobility and happiness.

2.2 Exercises to Support Bone Health

Maintaining and improving bone density becomes paramount as we age, particularly given the susceptibility to osteoporosis. Bone-strengthening exercises are critical in preserving bone health. Among these, weight-bearing exercises, which require you to work against gravity while supporting your weight, are especially beneficial. They stimulate bone formation and slow the rate of bone loss, effectively combating the natural decline in bone density that accompanies aging. Certain types of chair yoga, like standing from a seated position or using light weights, can be adapted to function as weight-bearing exercises, thereby contributing to bone health. Engaging in these exercises regularly can significantly reduce the risk of osteoporosis-related fractures, a common concern for older adults. By strengthening bones through consistent practice, you improve your physical resilience and enhance your safety.

Incorporating specific chair yoga poses and standing exercises into your routine can substantially support bone health. Here are a few suggestions to get started.

Interactive Element:

This book includes these exercises in its chapters on strengthening. Adding weight to chair exercises helps strengthen bones and support bone health.

SEATED CHAIR PRESS:

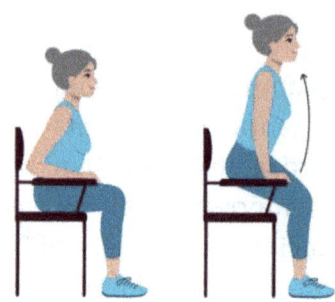

- Sit comfortably in the armchair, keeping your back straight.
- Place your hands on the armrests.
- Breathe in, and as you exhale, push down on the armrests to lift your body slightly off the chair. Try to lift your body using your arm strength more than pushing with your legs.
- Inhale and slowly lower yourself to the seated position.
- Perform 5-10 repetitions and do 2-4 sets.

CHAIR PLANK:

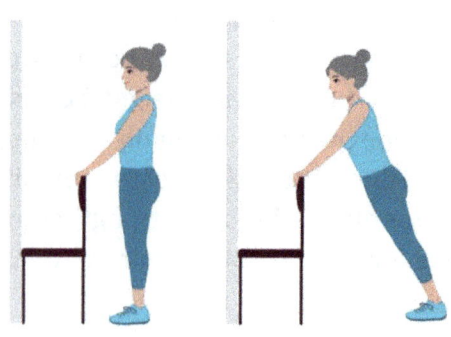

- Brace the chair against something sturdy, so it will not move.
- Place your hands on the back of the chair with your elbows straight.
- Extend your legs back one at a time. Your body should form a straight line from your head to your heels.
- Hold for a count of 5, then return to standing.
- Perform 5 repetitions and do 2-4 sets.

CHAIR PLANK-Modification:

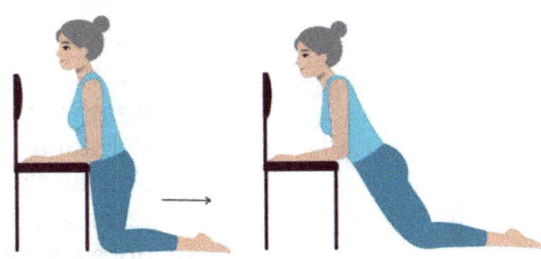

- Kneel in front of the chair; place your forearms on the chair's seat, elbows directly under your shoulders.
- Extend your legs back one at a time. Your body should form a straight line from your head to your knees.
- Hold for a count of 5, then return to a relaxed position.
- Perform 5 repetitions, and do 2-4 sets.

CHAIR PLANK-Progression:

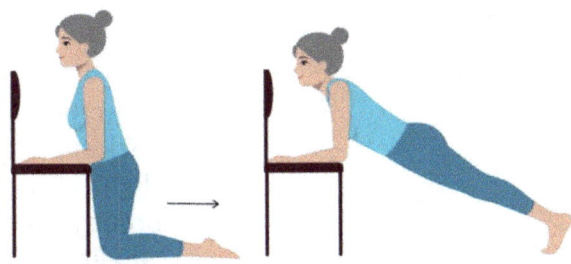

- Kneel in front of the chair, then place your hands or forearms on the chair's seat, elbows directly under your shoulders.
- Extend your legs back one at a time. Your hips should be down, and your body should form a straight line from your head to your heels.
- Hold for a count of 5, then return to a relaxed position.
- Perform 5 repetitions and do 2-4 sets.

CHAIR SQUAT:

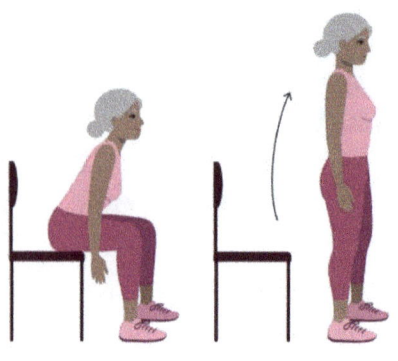

- Sit on the edge of the chair, feet hip-width apart.
- Breathe in, then exhale, and stand up. Use your arms on the chair if necessary, but try to rely more on your leg muscles.
- Inhale and lower yourself back into the chair. Use your arms if needed.
- Perform 5-10 repetitions and do 2-4 sets.
- For added resistance, hold water bottles or weighted bags.

SEATED MARCHING:

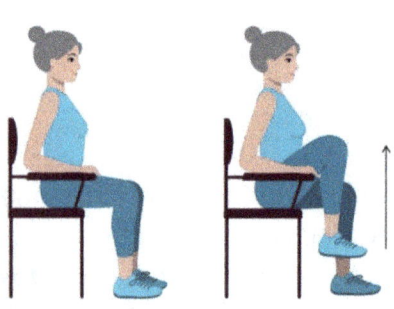

- Sit in the chair with your back supported or slightly forward.
- Breathe in and exhale as you lift your right knee towards your chest as high as comfortably. Inhale and gently lower your leg back down.
- Repeat the motion with the other leg.
- Perform 10-15 repetitions and 2-4 sets.
- You can use ankle weights for resistance.

Safety remains a top priority, especially for seniors with osteoporosis. Ensuring proper alignment throughout these exercises is crucial to avoid unnecessary strain on your bones and joints. When practicing weight-bearing exercises, focus on maintaining a neutral spine and ensuring correct alignment of your hips, knees, and ankles. This alignment not only prevents injury but also maximizes the effectiveness of each exercise.

Bone health is about preventing fractures and sustaining an active and independent lifestyle. Incorporating weight-bearing exercises into your routine can help mitigate the natural loss of bone density, promoting stronger, healthier bones.

2.3 Improving Cardiovascular Health with Chair Yoga

As we age, our heart's capacity to pump blood efficiently can decline, leading to increased risks of heart disease. However, incorporating chair yoga into your routine can help mitigate these risks by reducing blood pressure and cholesterol levels. A comprehensive review of 64 randomized controlled trials, detailed in "Yoga: A Flexible Way to Enhance Heart Health," found significant improvements in cardiovascular markers among yoga practitioners. On average, systolic blood pressure decreased by 4.5 points, and LDL cholesterol dropped by 7.6 points. These findings highlight how chair yoga's gentle approach can effectively support heart health without the strain of high-impact exercises.

Interactive Element:

These exercises, along with others, are included in the cardiovascular section of this book. Here are a few to get you started.

Use a low or no weight as a starting point and perform these exercises quickly, aiming for at least one repetition every second. Sustain the movement as long as possible, aiming for between 30 and 60 seconds of sustained movement, and do 3 to 5 repetitions.

CHAIR AEROBICS:

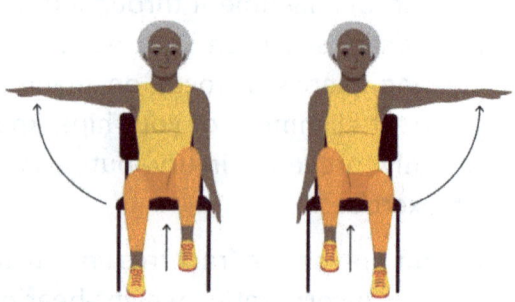

- Sit at the edge of your chair with your back straight and your hands resting at your sides.
- Alternate raising your right arm out to the side to shoulder height while lifting your left knee towards your chest, then switch to the left arm and right knee.
- Keep this movement brisk but controlled, aiming for coordination between arm and leg movements.

CHAIR RUNNING:

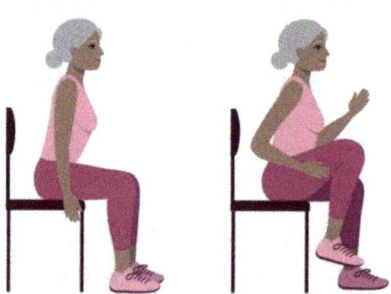

- Lean forward slightly in your chair, ensuring your feet are flat on the floor and your back is not too far from the backrest for support if needed.
- Begin by lifting your knees alternately as if you're jogging in place.
- Keep the movements quick and rhythmic, simulating running without leaving the seat.

PUNCH AND KICK COMBO:

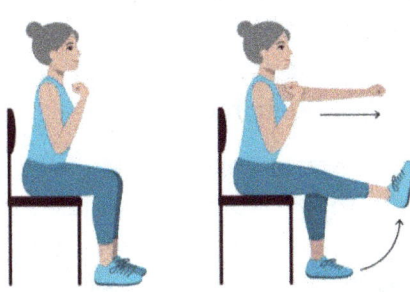

- ○ Lean forward slightly in your chair, keeping your back close to the backrest for support if needed.
- ○ Alternate punching forward with each arm while doing kicks with the opposite leg, such as, punching with your right arm as you kick with your left leg, then switch.
- ○ Keep the movements controlled but as fast as comfortably possible.

Consistency is the key to unlocking the full cardiovascular benefits of chair yoga. Regular practice can help strengthen the heart and improve overall circulation, which is essential for maintaining a healthy cardiovascular system. Establishing a daily or weekly routine ensures that your heart continues to reap the rewards of chair cardio exercises. Gradual progression is also crucial, allowing you to increase speed, repetitions, and sets as your heart strengthens and your endurance improves. By committing to regular practice, you can create a stable environment for cardiovascular improvement, reducing the risks associated with heart disease and high blood pressure.

2.4 Managing and Maintaining Weight with Chair Exercises

Chair exercises, including chair cardio, offer numerous benefits for weight loss in seniors. These activities are particularly advantageous because they are low-impact, reducing the risk of injury while providing an effective workout.

Maintaining or losing weight can be challenging for seniors due to reduced metabolic rates and mobility issues. Still, chair exercises can help by increasing heart rate and burning calories without standing or walking. Regular participation in chair cardio can enhance cardiovascular health, boosting circulation and oxygenation throughout the body and aiding metabolism.

Moreover, these exercises engage multiple muscle groups, helping preserve muscle mass that naturally declines with age. This muscle preservation can lead to a higher basal metabolic rate, meaning more calories are burned even at rest. Additionally, chair exercises improve flexibility and balance, contributing to overall physical function and independence, which motivates seniors to stay active.

Weight loss achieved through such exercises can also lead to reduced joint stress, better management of conditions like diabetes, and an overall improvement in quality of life.

2.5 Connecting Exercise with Improved Mental Health

The benefits of regular exercise, including chair yoga, are profound and far-reaching in mental health. Engaging in physical activity releases endorphins, the body's natural mood elevators. These biochemical reactions play a crucial role in alleviating symptoms of depression and anxiety, fostering a sense of well-being and emotional resilience. For many seniors, finding a form of exercise that is both accessible and enjoyable can significantly enhance mental health. Chair yoga, with its gentle approach, offers just that. The rhythmic movements and focused breathing promote relaxation, reducing stress and anxiety levels. As a result, practitioners often experience improved sleep patterns, another critical component of mental health. Regular chair yoga supports the physical body and nurtures the mind, creating a harmonious balance that enhances overall well-being.

Chair yoga includes specific exercises to calm the mind and soothe the nervous system, improving mental clarity and promoting relaxation. Seated meditation is a cornerstone of this practice, inviting you to sit quietly and focus on your breath. This simple act of mindfulness shifts attention away from stressors, grounding you in the present moment. Deep breathing exercises complement meditation, encouraging slow, deliberate breaths that foster relaxation. These techniques serve as powerful tools for stress relief, promoting a mindful approach to life's challenges. Visualization exercises also play a role, guiding the mind to imagine serene landscapes or calming scenarios. This mental imagery helps to quiet the mind, releasing tension and promoting tranquility. Together, these practices create a sanctuary of peace, supporting mental and emotional health.

Do not underestimate the social aspect of chair yoga. Participating in group yoga sessions or community classes enhances physical health and provides significant mental benefits. The shared experience of practicing yoga fosters a sense of community and belonging, which are vital components of mental well-being. Engaging with others in a supportive environment offers opportunities for building new friendships and connections and can alleviate feelings of isolation, a common concern among seniors. The encouragement and fellowship found within a yoga class can boost motivation and morale, reinforcing the positive effects of the practice.

Real-life examples often serve as powerful illustrations of chair yoga's impact on mental health. Consider the story of a senior woman living alone who was encouraged to join a chair yoga class at the community center because she felt overwhelmed by loneliness. She discovered that the class offered an upbeat environment with people her age. Over time, she reported a noticeable improvement in well-being, reduced loneliness, and a sense of belonging. Her focus and concentration also improved, allowing her to engage more fully in activities she once found daunting.

Similarly, another testament to chair yoga's benefits comes from a retired schoolteacher who found that chair yoga helped him navigate the challenges of depression. The structured routine provided a sense of purpose, while the social interaction of group classes lifted his spirits.

Both stories highlight how chair yoga can combat loneliness and depression, offering not just physical but profound emotional benefits. These testimonials underscore the transformative power of chair yoga in enhancing mental health, offering hope and inspiration for others seeking similar benefits. Join a class or encourage someone you know to try it; the potential for positive change is immense.

Chair yoga's ability to strengthen mental health is a testament to its holistic approach. Addressing the physical and emotional dimensions of well-being offers a comprehensive path to improved health. As you practice, you nurture your body and cultivate a more resilient and balanced mind. Integrating physical movement, mindful breathing, and social interaction creates a rich tapestry of support, empowering you to thrive in all aspects of life.

In this chapter, we've explored how chair yoga addresses common health challenges. The next chapter will delve into nutrition and hydration, two vital components of an active and healthy lifestyle. Focusing on protein consumption and fluid intake, we will reveal how these elements complement your exercise routine, supporting strength, endurance, and overall vitality.

Chapter 3: Nutrition and Hydration for Optimal Performance

Oftentimes, patients tell me about their struggles with fatigue and muscle weakness. Despite enthusiasm for daily walks, exercise, and commitment to staying active, they find it increasingly challenging to complete their routines. I hear these complaints frequently from aging adults; it highlights a critical component of senior health—nutrition. After reviewing their diet, it became clear that protein intake was insufficient, a common issue many seniors face. After educating them to make a few dietary adjustments, they soon experienced a resurgence of energy and strength. This chapter will explore the crucial role of nutrition and hydration in maintaining energy, particularly the importance of protein in muscle health.

3.1 Protein Power: Building Muscles and Tissues

Protein is the building block for muscle health and is pivotal in muscle repair and growth. As we age, maintaining muscle mass becomes increasingly vital. Protein supports the body's natural repair processes, aiding recovery from daily wear and tear. Essential amino acids, the building blocks of protein, are particularly crucial in this process, stimulating muscle protein synthesis and helping preserve muscle mass. Sarcopenia, a condition characterized by losing muscle mass and function, poses a significant threat to independence among seniors, making adequate protein consumption essential.

Protein-calorie malnutrition in seniors significantly impacts their ability to build or maintain muscle mass. This condition arises when dietary protein intake falls below what the body requires, which can be due to factors such as reduced appetite, dental issues, or chronic health conditions. Insufficient protein consumption exacerbates the natural diminishment of muscle mass with age. Inadequate protein intake impairs muscle protein synthesis, leading to muscle wasting. Additionally, a lack of caloric intake forces the body to break down muscle tissue for energy, accelerating muscle loss. This compromises mobility and strength, increases pain levels and fall risk, diminishes metabolic rate, and can lead to a vicious cycle of inactivity and further weakness.

Several risk factors contribute to malnutrition among seniors. These include a diminished appetite, difficulty chewing or swallowing, and limited access to nutritious foods. Certain medical conditions and medications can also exacerbate nutritional deficiencies. To combat these challenges, regular dietary assessments by healthcare providers can identify and address malnutrition early. Incorporating nutrient-dense snacks between meals can also help maintain adequate calorie and protein intake.

High-quality protein sources are essential for seniors. Lean meats such as chicken, turkey, and fish offer excellent options, rich in essential amino acids. Boiled eggs and plant-based proteins, including walnuts, pecans, and pistachios, make nutritious protein snacks. Protein drinks and bars can serve as convenient supplements, ensuring adequate daily protein intake. Dairy products like milk, cheese, and yogurt offer additional sources of high-quality protein suitable for incorporating into various meals.

Experts emphasize the importance of determining the protein intake needed to meet health and fitness goals. While the Recommended Dietary Allowance (RDA) sets protein at 0.8 grams per kilogram (or approximately 0.36 grams per pound) of body weight per day, experts suggest that seniors should aim for 1.2 to 2.0 grams per kilogram (or about 0.54 to 0.91 grams per pound) to maintain muscle health effectively. Seniors should balance this increased protein intake with other macronutrients, such as unsaturated fats like olive oil and avocado, and carbohydrates such as fruits and whole grains to support overall health comprehensively. The "even distribution hypothesis" advocates for seniors to spread their protein intake evenly across meals to enhance muscle mass preservation in this demographic.

Incorporating protein into daily meals need not be complex. Simple adjustments can make a significant difference. Starting the day with protein-rich foods like eggs instead of cereal can set a positive tone for nutritional intake. Throughout the day, snacking on walnuts, pecans, almonds, or a protein bar can provide a steady source of protein. Including a protein source in every meal, whether lean meat, dairy products, or plant-based alternatives, is crucial. These strategies ensure protein intake supports muscle health, increasing overall strength and energy.

3.2 Hydration Essentials: Preventing Dehydration

Hydration supports various bodily functions. As we age, maintaining adequate hydration becomes increasingly vital. Water is a component of joint lubrication, helping to maintain smooth movement and reduce discomfort. It regulates body temperature, dissipates heat, and maintains a stable internal environment. Moreover, proper hydration ensures efficient digestion, nutrient absorption, and waste elimination. These processes collectively enhance exercise performance, enabling seniors to engage in physical activities with greater ease and endurance. Water supports cardiovascular health by aiding in blood pressure regulation, reducing heart strain during exercise, and preventing dizziness caused by too low blood pressure.

Recognizing the signs of dehydration is crucial in preventing potential health complications. Dehydration can manifest subtly, yet its effects can be profound.

- Dry Mouth - A dry mouth and persistent fatigue indicate that your body lacks sufficient fluids.
- Dizziness - As dehydration progresses, dizziness may occur, often signaling a drop in blood pressure. This dizziness can lead to instability, increasing the risk of falls and injuries.
- Dark Yellow Urine - Dark yellow urine is a visible indicator, suggesting concentrated waste products resulting from insufficient water intake.
- Skin Turgor – This refers to the skin's elasticity, or its ability to quickly return to its normal shape after being gently pinched and released. When you pinch the skin and let go, well-hydrated skin snaps back immediately. If it takes longer to flatten out, it may indicate dehydration or reduced elasticity, which can occur with age, illness, or poor nutrition.

Skin turgor can be a useful indicator of fluid status in seniors, although it becomes less reliable as the skin naturally loses some elasticity over time. For example, dehydrated skin may feel doughy or sluggish to recover, whereas healthy, hydrated skin feels firm and resilient. It's not a standalone diagnostic tool—it's often paired with other signs, such as dry mouth or dizziness—but it's a quick, non-invasive check that anyone can observe.

Awareness of these symptoms allows you to take proactive measures, such as addressing dehydration before it escalates into more severe health issues.

For seniors, the guidelines for daily water intake can vary significantly based on individual health, activity level, and environmental conditions. The current U.S. National Academies of Sciences, Engineering, and Medicine recommendations suggest that an adequate daily fluid intake for older adults should generally be around 1.7 liters (approximately 7 cups) for women and slightly higher for men. However, these figures include fluids from all sources, not just water. You can adjust this based on factors such as physical activity, where you may need to increase intake to account for sweat loss, or specific health conditions, such as kidney or heart disease, which may necessitate fluid restrictions under medical advice. Tailoring hydration to one's unique health profile ensures optimal well-being.

Maintaining adequate hydration throughout the day can be achieved through practical strategies. Setting reminders to drink water at regular intervals can help establish a routine, ensuring consistent fluid intake. Using marked water bottles provides a visual cue, enabling you to track your consumption and adjust as needed. This tool can be particularly useful in reinforcing hydration habits, as it provides a tangible measure of progress. For those who find plain water unappealing, adding natural flavorings such as slices of lemon, cucumber, or berries can enhance the taste, making it more enjoyable.

Consider pairing water intake with routine activities, such as drinking water before each meal or after using the restroom. This approach integrates hydration into existing habits, reducing the likelihood of forgetting to drink. Additionally, consuming foods with high water content, such as celery, cucumbers, and oranges, can help supplement fluid intake while providing essential nutrients. This strategy supports hydration while enhancing your diet with vitamins and minerals. By incorporating these practices into your daily routine, you can maintain optimal hydration levels, which in turn support your overall health.

3.3 Nutritional Tips for Enhanced Energy Levels

Understanding the connection between nutrition and energy is paramount in maintaining vitality and vigor, especially as we age. Carbohydrates are essential for energy production, serving as the body's primary fuel source. Cells use glucose, produced when the body converts carbohydrates, to generate energy. This process is essential for fueling both physical activity and mental functions. However, not all carbohydrates are created equal. Complex carbohydrates in whole grains and certain vegetables release energy slowly, providing a steady and sustained fuel source. This gradual release helps maintain consistent energy levels throughout the day, preventing the spikes and crashes associated with simple sugars. Incorporating these carbohydrates into your diet can help you engage in daily activities with greater ease and endurance.

Supplements and vitamins can also play a role in boosting energy, especially when dietary intake falls short. While a balanced diet should provide most of the necessary nutrients, supplements can help fill gaps, particularly if you have specific deficiencies. Vitamins and minerals play significant roles in metabolic processes, contributing to energy production at the cellular level. For instance, B vitamins convert food into energy, supporting overall metabolic function. Vitamin D deficiency in adults is quite common and can significantly impact energy levels by reducing serotonin production, which affects mood and stamina. According to the National Institutes of Health, a significant portion of the adult population suffers from vitamin D insufficiency, which can potentially lead to fatigue and decreased energy. Minerals such as magnesium and iron are essential for maintaining energy levels, supporting muscle function, and facilitating oxygen transport.

Always consult a healthcare provider before adding supplements to your routine to make sure they align with your health needs and goals.

Ensuring an adequate intake of these nutrients is crucial, as deficiencies can lead to fatigue and reduced stamina. Fresh fruits and vegetables, rich in antioxidants, are excellent sources of these essential vitamins and minerals. They provide energy-boosting nutrients and help protect the body from oxidative stress, promoting overall health. By incorporating a variety of colorful fruits and vegetables into your meals, you can naturally boost your energy levels.

Consider adopting specific eating patterns and habits to maintain steady energy throughout the day. One effective strategy is consuming small, frequent meals rather than three large ones. This approach helps stabilize blood sugar levels, reducing the likelihood of energy dips. By providing your body with consistent nourishment, you ensure a continuous energy supply, enabling you to stay active and alert. Combining protein with complex carbohydrates at each meal further supports this goal. Protein helps slow the digestion of carbohydrates, leading to a more gradual release of glucose. This combination of nutrients helps balance blood sugar levels and extends the duration of energy availability, thereby improving your stamina and endurance.

Preparing meals in advance can simplify this process, ensuring you have healthy options readily available. Additionally, pay attention to portion sizes and listen to your body's hunger cues; eat when you feel hungry and stop when you're satisfied. By fostering a balanced and varied diet, you can support your body's energy needs, enhancing your ability to enjoy daily activities.

3.4 Nutritional Tips for Post-Exercise Recovery

The period immediately after exercise is critical for recovery and muscle repair. You need to replenish the energy stores depleted during physical activity after your workout. Exercise causes your muscles to undergo stress and experience minor damage, a natural part of the strengthening and adaptation process. Consuming nutrients after exercise helps repair this damage, enabling your body to rebuild muscles that are stronger and more resilient. The role of carbohydrates in restoring glycogen levels is significant, as they replenish the energy stores used during your workout. Meanwhile, proteins help repair and build muscle tissue, aiming to preserve muscle mass. Ensuring your body receives the proper nutrients promptly after exercise can enhance recovery, reduce soreness, and prepare you for your next activity.

Optimal recovery foods should focus on high-quality proteins and healthy fats to support the rebuilding process. Protein sources, such as protein drinks, protein bars, and lean meats, are excellent for building and maintaining muscle. These foods provide the essential amino acids necessary for repairing muscle fibers and promoting growth. Additionally, avocados are a beneficial source of healthy fats and potassium, an electrolyte vital for maintaining fluid balance and preventing muscle cramps. Incorporating seasonal fruits into your post-exercise meal provides a natural source of carbohydrates and vitamins, offering sustained energy and supporting recovery. These fruits, rich in antioxidants, also help reduce inflammation, further supporting recovery. A balanced approach that includes these elements can significantly enhance your post-exercise nutrition.

Timing your post-exercise meal correctly maximizes its benefits. Ideally, you should consume a meal or snack within 30 to 60 minutes after exercising. This timing enhances your body's absorption of nutrients, leading to more efficient recovery. By planning your meals around your exercise schedule, you can ensure that your body receives the necessary nutrients during this optimal period, thereby enhancing the effectiveness of your workout regimen.

Hydration is another essential component of post-exercise recovery. During exercise, your body loses fluids through sweat; rehydrating is necessary to restore balance. Drinking water or electrolyte-rich drinks helps replenish lost fluids and electrolytes, which are crucial for regulating nerve and muscle function. Monitoring fluid intake after exercise ensures that your body remains optimally hydrated, supporting all physiological processes involved in recovery. Adequate rehydration reduces the risk of cramping and fatigue, allowing you to recover more quickly and efficiently. Staying hydrated actively maintains cognitive function and keeps overall energy levels up, which dehydration can diminish.

Incorporating these nutritional strategies into your routine can significantly enhance your recovery and support your short-term and long-term fitness goals. Focusing on balanced nutrition and proper hydration provides your body with the necessary tools to repair, rebuild, and thrive after exercise. Attention to post-exercise nutrition underscores the holistic approach to health and wellness, integrating physical activity with mindful eating and hydration practices. With these insights, you can support your body's recovery and continue to improve health and stamina.

As we conclude this chapter, the information shared emphasizes the vital role nutrition and hydration play in sustaining physical and mental health. The critical integration of nutrition and exercise fosters a comprehensive approach to building strength and improving endurance.

The next chapter will delve into practical exercise routines, offering step-by-step guidance on enhancing overall strength and improving balance through chair yoga.

Chapter 4: Building Strength Through Chair Exercises

Some of the most inspiring stories begin with simple resources for home workouts. Consider a retired school teacher whose upper body strength had been waning, making tasks like lifting shopping bags or reaching high shelves challenging. As her physical therapist, I introduced her to chair exercises and incorporated water bottles and weighted grocery bags for resistance. Over time, her strength improved, enabling her to handle daily activities more easily. Her experience exemplifies how regular, focused exercise can transform one's quality of life. She sidestepped the cost of gym equipment by utilizing everyday household items, proving that effective fitness solutions can be both accessible and practical. This story highlights the potential within each of us to reclaim our strength and independence, a central theme of this chapter.

4.1 Upper Body Strengthening

Upper body strength training is not merely about lifting weights or building muscle mass; it is about enhancing your capacity to navigate daily life easily and confidently. Stronger arms and shoulders contribute significantly to your ability to perform essential activities. Whether carrying groceries, opening jars, or lifting grandchildren into your arms, these tasks become more manageable with increased upper body strength. Moreover, as you build strength, you may notice an improvement in your posture. Stronger muscles support your spine, reducing the likelihood of back and neck strain and discomfort often accompanying poor posture. This alignment contributes to physical well-being and enhances your overall appearance and confidence.

Incorporating water bottles and bags with handles into your exercise routine offers a practical and accessible approach to strength training. These everyday items serve as useful tools for resistance exercises. By filling water bottles to a comfortable weight or using a sturdy grocery bag filled with items, you can perform various arm exercises, such as bicep curls and overhead presses. The added weight provides the resistance needed to challenge your muscles, encouraging growth and resilience. This versatility allows you to adjust the difficulty of your workouts as your strength improves, ensuring continuous progress.

Engaging in regular upper-body strength training not only improves physical capabilities but also enhances endurance. As you strengthen your muscles, you increase their ability to sustain prolonged activity without fatigue. This endurance is crucial for maintaining energy levels throughout the day, enabling you to participate in activities you enjoy without feeling exhausted. Whether it's gardening, performing household chores, or participating in community events, a strong upper body supports your active lifestyle.

For those new to upper-body strength training, it is essential to start with exercises that match your current fitness level. Start with either lighter or no weight and focus on mastering proper form. This foundation ensures that you perform exercises safely, minimizing the risk of injury. As your confidence and strength grow, gradually increase the weight or resistance, challenging your muscles to adapt and improve. Consistency is key to reaping the full benefits of strength training. Aim to incorporate these exercises into your routine several times a week, allowing time for rest and recovery between sessions. This balanced approach supports muscle growth and endurance while preventing overuse injuries.

Interactive Element: Upper Body Exercises

Consider using the following checklist to help you incorporate upper-body chair exercises into your routine. This tool enables you to track your exercises, ensuring a comprehensive workout that targets all major muscle groups. By checking off each exercise as you complete it, you can monitor your progress and maintain motivation.

Incorporate the following breathing technique with each exercise: Exhale during the lifting phase of each exercise. This can help support the spine and prevent a sudden increase in blood pressure. Inhale during the lowering phase of each exercise. This helps stabilize your core and prepare for the next lift.

Start with less resistance than you think you can handle, or no resistance at all, to prevent overstressing your tendons and muscles. Once this exercise becomes easy, you can increase the number of repetitions and/or sets or add weight. Most importantly, move your joints within a pain-free range of motion.

BICEP CURLS: Purpose- Strengthens the biceps, which can help with tasks like lifting objects or opening doors. Try using water bottles, weighted bags, elastic bands, or dumbbells for resistance.

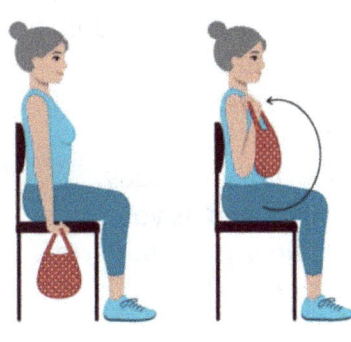

- Sit on a chair with your back supported, arms extended down by your sides.
- Breathe in and exhale as you bend your elbow towards your shoulder. Only your forearms should move. Avoid swinging or using momentum.
- As you inhale, slowly lower the weight back to the starting position.
- Perform 10-15 reps and 2-4 sets.

OVERHEAD PRESS: Purpose- Targets the shoulders and triceps, which aid in reaching overhead or pushing objects. Try using water bottles or dumbbells for resistance.

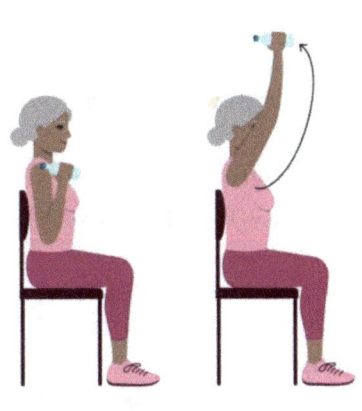

- Sit on a chair with your back supported. Bend your elbow and hold your hands at shoulder height, palms facing each other.
- Breathe in, and slowly press upwards as you exhale. Extend your arm until it's as straight as comfortably possible.
- Keep your neck relaxed and gaze forward, not up at the bottle.
- Inhale and gently lower your hands to shoulder level.
- Perform 10-15 reps and 2-4 sets.

LATERAL ARM RAISES: Purpose- Strengthens muscles on the side of the shoulders, helping with movements like dressing or reaching sideways. Try using water bottles, weighted bags, or dumbbells for resistance.

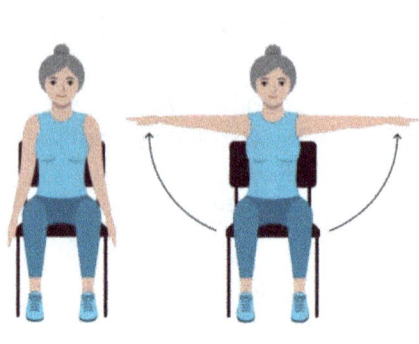

- Sit on a chair with your back supported, arms extended down by your sides.
- Hold the weights at your sides (or just your arms), palms facing your body.
- Breathe in, and as you exhale, slowly lift your arms to the sides as high as is comfortable.
- Inhale and slowly lower the arms back to your sides, maintaining control.
- Perform 10-15 reps and 2-4 sets.

FRONT ARM RAISES: Purpose- Strengthens muscles in front of the shoulders, helping with reaching and lifting. Try using water bottles, weighted bags, or dumbbells for resistance.

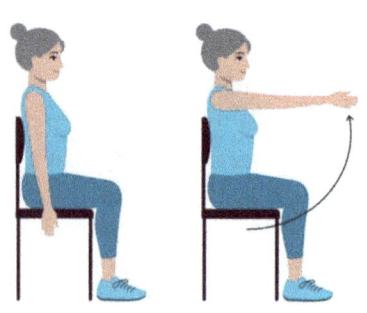

- Sit on a chair with your back supported, arms extended down by your sides.
- Hold the weights at your sides (or just your arms), palms facing your body.
- Breathe in, and as you exhale, slowly lift your arms up as high as is comfortable.
- Inhale and slowly lower your arms back to your sides, maintaining control.
- Perform 10-15 reps and 2-4 sets.

SHOULDER AND TRICEP EXTENSIONS: <u>Purpose</u> - Improves the strength of the triceps and stability of the shoulders, assisting with pushing movements or extending arms backward. Try using water bottles, weighted bags, or dumbbells for resistance

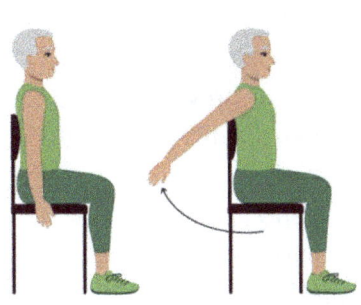

- Sit on a chair with your back supported. Hold the weights at your sides (or just use your arms), palms facing your body.
- Breathe in, and as you exhale, extend your arms backward, keeping them straight or with a slight elbow bend.
- Breathe in as you slowly bring your arms back to your sides.
- Perform 10-15 reps and 2-4 sets.

SEATED CHAIR PRESS: <u>Purpose</u> - Works the chest, shoulders, and triceps, increasing upper body strength for tasks that require pushing or lifting. Use a chair with armrests.

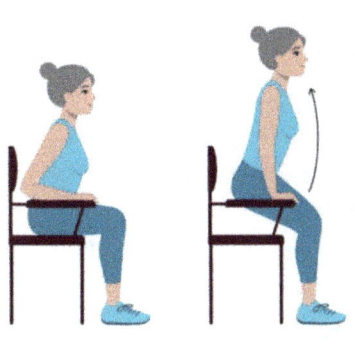

- Sit on a chair, ensuring your back is not resting against the chair, and lean slightly forward with your hands on the armrests.
- Breathe in, and as you exhale, push down on the armrests to lift your body slightly off the chair. (Don't worry if you cannot lift your body fully off the chair.)
- Try to lift your body using your arm strength more than pushing with your legs.
- Inhale and slowly lower yourself to the seated position.
- Perform 10-15 reps and 2-4 sets.

WRIST AND FOREARM STRENGTHENING: <u>Purpose</u> - Enhances grip strength and wrist stability for activities like writing or holding utensils. Try using water bottles, weighted bags, or dumbbells for resistance. Do both wrists at the same time or alternate them.

Wrist Curls:

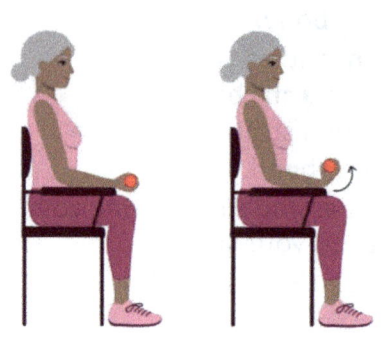

- Sit on a chair with your back supported.
- Rest your forearm on the arms of your chair or on your thigh, palm facing up, with the weight in your hand.
- Breathe in and curl your wrist upward as you exhale. Only the wrist should move.
- Inhale as you slowly lower the weight down.
- Perform 10-15 reps and 2-4 sets.

Reverse Wrist Curls:

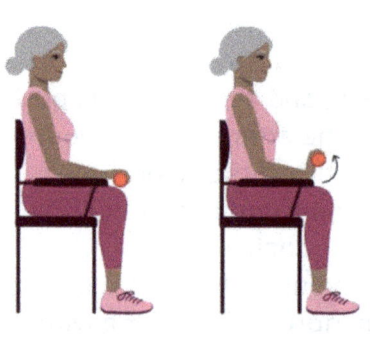

- Sit on a chair with your back supported.
- Rest your forearm on the arms of your chair or on your thigh, palm facing down, with the weight in your hand.
- Breathe in and curl your wrist upward as you exhale. Only the wrist should move.
- Inhale as you slowly lower the weight down.
- Perform 10-15 reps and 2-4 sets.

CHEST OPENER: Purpose - To strengthen shoulder, upper back, and arm muscles, improving posture, better breathing, and arm movement. Try using water bottles or dumbbells for resistance.

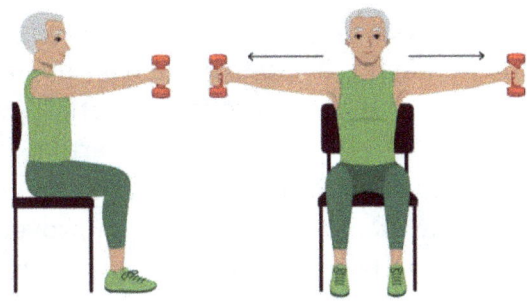

- Sit with your back supported or slightly forward.
- Hold your arms extended forward at chest height, palms facing each other.
- Breathe in, and as you exhale, open your arms to the sides, squeeze your shoulder blades together. The movement should resemble opening a book.
- Inhale as you bring your arms back together.
- Perform 10-15 reps and 2-4 sets.

    This checklist offers a structured approach to your workouts, ensuring you engage in a balanced and effective upper-body routine. By consistently tracking your exercises, you can identify areas for improvement and celebrate achievements, reinforcing your commitment to building strength and independence.

    Upper body strength training is more than a physical exercise; it is a pathway to enhanced independence and improved quality of life. As you embrace this practice, you empower yourself to tackle daily challenges with confidence and ease. Whether through water bottles, grocery bags, or other household items, the tools for building strength are within reach. Embrace the opportunity to strengthen your body and enrich your life through the transformative power of exercise.

4.2 Lower Body Strengthening

A 75-year-old retiree had been grappling with balance issues and difficulty standing up from a chair following a hip fracture, compounded by a sedentary lifestyle that left his leg muscles weak. He began a chair yoga exercise program focused on strengthening his legs to regain his independence. I gradually advanced him to standing exercises as his leg muscles improved. Starting with supported standing poses that utilize a chair or countertop for balance, he progressed to free-standing exercises, such as gentle squats and standing leg lifts. This transition markedly improved his strength, balance, and confidence. He could stand up from his chair more easily and walk with a steadier gait, embracing daily activities with renewed vigor and self-assurance.

Lower body strength is the cornerstone of maintaining mobility and independence as we age. Strong legs support your body, providing a solid foundation for everyday activities such as walking, climbing stairs, and standing for extended periods. Strong leg muscles also play a pivotal role in reducing the risk of falls, a common and profound concern for older adults. By strengthening the muscles that support balance and stability, you reduce the risk of stumbling or losing your balance, creating a safer and more secure environment for yourself.

A chair can be a valuable tool in performing lower body exercises safely, offering support and stability as you strengthen your legs. If your budget allows, resistance bands and ankle weights are excellent items to have on hand for strengthening your legs. If not, you can use household objects for resistance training. For example, you can grab a pair of long socks, fill them with rice or beans, secure the ends, and use these as ankle weights. Strong, thick, elastic waistbands cut from unused shorts or pants also make good resistance bands.

Interactive Element: Lower Body Exercises

Consider using the following checklist to help you incorporate lower-body chair exercises into your routine. This tool enables you to track your exercises, ensuring a comprehensive workout that targets all major muscle groups. By checking off each exercise as you complete it, you can monitor your progress and maintain motivation.

Remember to use the breathing technique outlined in the upper body section: Exhale during the lifting phase of each exercise to help support the spine and prevent a sudden increase in blood pressure. Inhale during the lowering phase of each exercise to stabilize your core and prepare for the next lift.

Start with less resistance than you think you can handle, or no resistance, to prevent overstressing your tendons and muscles. Once this exercise becomes easy, you can increase the number of repetitions and/or sets or add weight. Most importantly, move your joints within a pain-free range.

SEATED LEG LIFT: Purpose- Strengthens the quadriceps and improves mobility, aiding in activities like standing from a seated position and walking. Try using ankle weights for resistance.

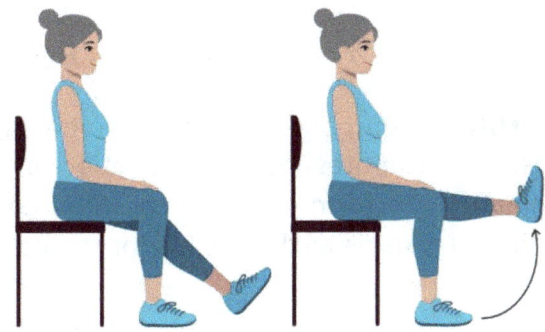

- Sit in the middle of the chair to allow room for leg movement.
- Rest one foot flat on the floor and extend the knee of the other leg, placing the heel on the floor.
- Take a deep breath and exhale as you lift the extended leg off the ground, keeping the knee straight but not locked. Lift as high as comfortably.
- Inhale and lower your leg back down.
- Do this on both legs. Perform 10-15 repetitions and 2-4 sets.

CHAIR SQUAT: Purpose- Strengthens the muscles of the legs while working the core for balance. It's crucial for leg strength and enhancing the ability to stand and sit. Try holding water bottles, weights, or weighted bags.

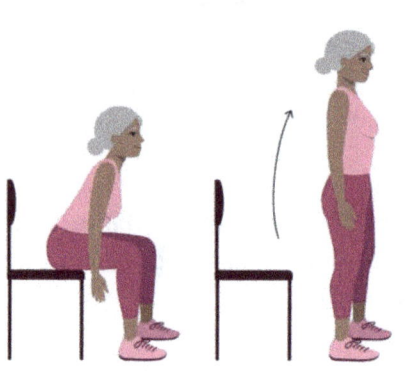

- Sit with your feet hip-width apart, leaning slightly forward.
- . Breathe in and exhale as you engage your core and push up through your heels to stand up. Use your arm strength on the chair, if necessary, but try to rely on your leg muscles.
- Inhale and slowly lower yourself back down. Perform 5-10 times and 2-4 sets.

SEATED MARCHING: Purpose- Strengthens the hip flexors and quadriceps muscles. Promotes better circulation in the legs and improves coordination. Perform on both legs. Alternate marching or do one leg at a time. Try using ankle weights for resistance

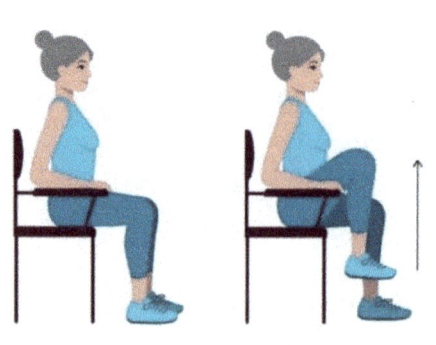

- Sit with your back supported or slightly forward.
- Lift your right knee towards your chest as high as comfortably.
- Gently lower your leg back to the starting position.
- Repeat the motion with the other leg and alternate legs, doing 10-15 lifts per leg. Repeat 2–3 sets.

SEATED KICKS: Purpose- Strengthens the quadriceps, the large muscles at the front of the thigh. Works on leg extension, helpful for walking, climbing stairs, and knee stability. Perform this exercise on both legs. You can alternate them or do one at a time. Try using ankle weights for resistance.

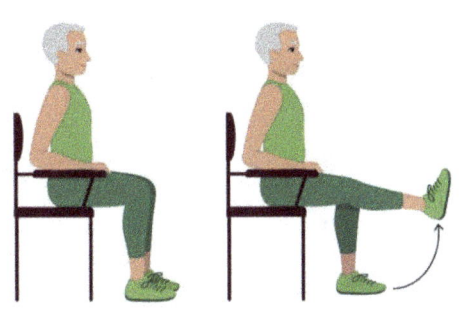

- Sit with your back supported or slightly forward.
- Breathe in and exhale as you extend one knee as straight as is comfortable. Your foot can be up or pointed.
- Inhale and lower your leg back down.
- Perform 10-15 repetitions and 2-4 sets.

INNER THIGH SQUEEZE: Purpose- Strengthens the muscles of the inner thighs. Improves stability when standing or walking, and helps with bringing legs together or sitting cross-legged. Use a pillow or rolled towel for resistance.

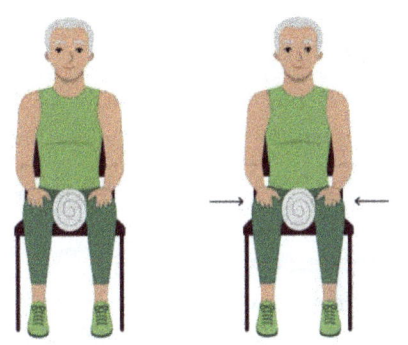

- Sit with your back supported or slightly forward.
- Place a pillow or rolled towel between your knees.
- Breath in and as you exhale, gently squeeze the pillow or towel with your knees.
- Squeeze for three to five seconds.
- Inhale and slowly release the squeeze.
- Perform 10-15 repetitions and 2-4 sets.

LEG OPEN/CLOSE: Purpose- This exercise targets the outer thigh muscles (abductors), promoting leg strength, enhancing hip mobility, and improving balance. Try using a resistance band around the thighs.

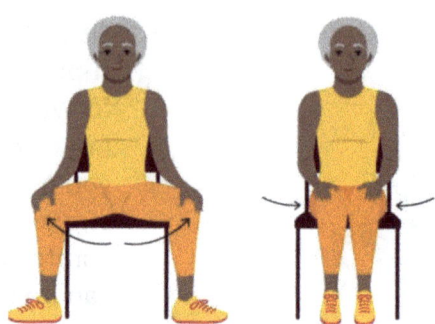

- Sit with your back supported or slightly forward.
- Begin with your knees together.
- Breathe in, and as you exhale, open your legs by moving your knees apart.
- Focus on using the outer thigh muscles. Open as wide as comfortably.
- Inhale and bring your knees back together.
- Perform 10-15 repetitions and do 2-4 sets.

Progression

- Utilizing resistance or weight, straighten the knee of 1 leg, keeping the other leg bent and the foot flat on the ground.
- Place the heel of the straightened leg on the ground.
- Using the outer thigh muscles, slide your heel to the side as far as possible without straining and then slide it back to the starting position.
- Perform 10-15 repetitions and do 2-4 sets.
- Repeat the motion on the other leg.

SEATED TOE RAISES: Purpose- Strengthens the muscles in the front of the lower leg and improves ankle mobility, and assists balance

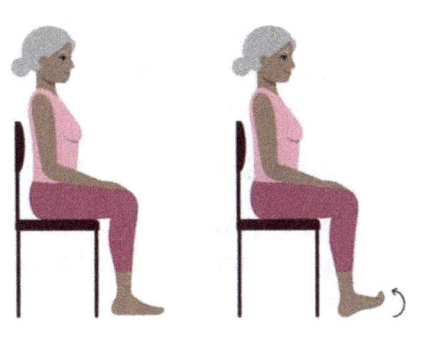

- ○ Sit with your back supported or slightly forward.
- ○ Lift your foot towards your shins while keeping your heels on the ground.
- ○ Hold this position for a count of three to five seconds.
- ○ Lower your toes back to the floor.
- ○ . Perform 10-15 repetitions and do 2-4 sets.

SEATED HEEL RAISES: Purpose- Strengthens the calf muscles and supports ankle stability, and assists balance.

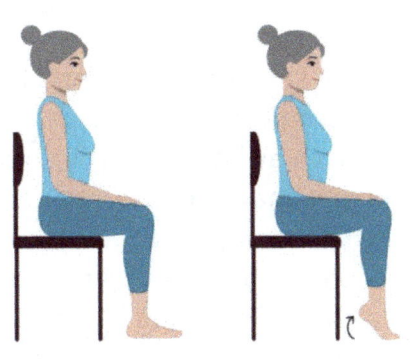

- ○ Sit with your back supported or slightly forward.
- ○ Lift your heels off the ground, balancing on the balls of your feet.
- ○ Hold this position for a count of three to five seconds.
- ○ Lower your heels back to the floor.
- ○ You can place a heavy book on your lap for resistance.
- ○ Perform 10-15 repetitions and do 2-4 sets.

Lower-body workouts are about more than muscle-building; they empower you to take control of your life. Incorporating these exercises into your routine strengthens your foundation, providing you with the confidence and stability to move freely. Think of the chair not just as a piece of equipment but as a symbol of support, helping you through movements that enhance your strength and sense of security.

4.3 Core Strength Exercises for Improved Balance

In the complex structure of the human body, the core serves as a foundational pillar, essential for maintaining balance and stability. Your core muscles play a crucial role in maintaining postural control and preventing falls. A strong core functions like a stabilizing belt, supporting the spine and pelvis, which are critical for maintaining an upright posture and affecting balance. This core stability ensures that your body remains steady during movement, significantly reducing the risk of falls and enhancing personal safety. We can compare the relationship between core strength and enhanced balance to the foundation of a building; just as a solid foundation supports an entire structure, a robust core supports your body's controlled movements with confidence and assurance.

The functional benefits of improved core strength manifest in various aspects of daily life. One of the most noticeable advantages is the ease of transitioning from a seated to a standing position, which requires a coordinated effort and stability. A strong core supports this action, making it smoother and less taxing on the body. This capability extends to household tasks, where tasks such as bending, lifting, and reaching become more manageable with enhanced core strength. Reducing back pain is another significant benefit, as a stable core alleviates pressure on the lower back, reducing the risk of strain and discomfort. Improved endurance is also a notable outcome, as a strong core supports prolonged activity without fatigue, enabling you to engage in activities with greater energy. Chair yoga offers a range of exercises specifically designed to target the core muscles, enhancing balance and stability.

Exercising tailored to your current fitness level is crucial for strengthening your core. Begin by focusing on engaging your abdominal muscles during movements, consciously tightening them to create a firm base. This engagement not only supports your spine but also enhances the effectiveness of each exercise. Breathing techniques are integral to core exercises, providing the rhythm and control needed to sustain effort. Inhale as you prepare for movement, and exhale as you engage your core, allowing the muscles to contract fully. This practice enhances muscle activation and promotes relaxation and focus, which are crucial for maintaining form and preventing strain.

Interactive Element: Core Exercises

Consider using the following checklist to help you incorporate core chair exercises into your routine. This tool enables you to track your exercises, ensuring a comprehensive workout that targets major muscle groups. By checking off each exercise as you complete it, you can monitor your progress and maintain motivation.

Remember to use the breathing technique outlined earlier: Inhale as you prepare for movement, and exhale as you engage your core, allowing the muscles to contract fully.to help support the spine.

You can also use resistance with these exercises. Start with less resistance than you think you can handle, or no resistance to prevent overstressing your tendons and muscles. Once this exercise becomes easy, you can increase the number of repetitions and/or sets or add weight. **Most importantly, move your joints within a pain-free range.**

CAUTION: Do not do twisting exercises if you have vertebral disc problems, a fused spine, or other conditions for which twisting is contraindicated. If you are unsure, please consult your physician.

SEATED TORSO TWIST: Purpose- Enhances spinal mobility and strengthens the obliques, which are crucial for reaching or bending to the side.

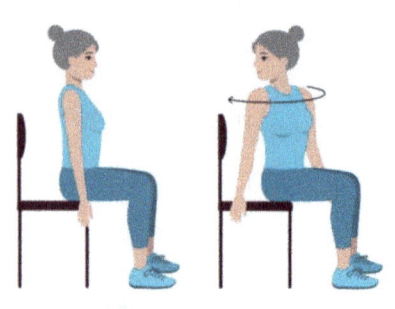

- Sit in the middle or at the edge of the chair.
- Cross your arms over your chest or hang your arms to the sides.
- Twist your upper body to one side, moving your head and shoulders together as if looking over your shoulder, keeping your hips facing forward.
- Do 10-15 repetitions and 2-4 sets, and repeat on the other side.

SEATED LEANING FRONT AND BACK: Purpose -Strengthens the abdominal and spinal muscles, promoting stability and balance.

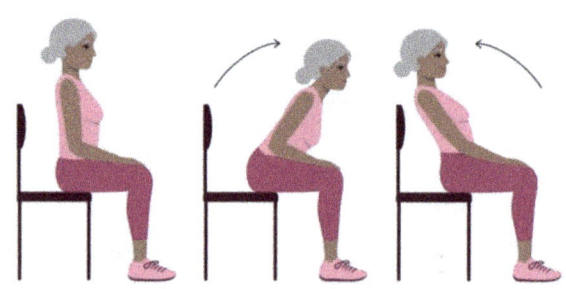

- Sit toward the edge of a chair with your hands on your thighs or crossed over your chest.
- Inhale, and as you exhale, lean your torso forward. Keep your back straight.
- Lean back as far as is comfortable.
- Move back and forth in a controlled manner.
- Do 10-15 repetitions and 2-4 sets.

SEATED SIDE REACHING: -Purpose- Strengthens the oblique muscles. This exercise improves lateral stability and enhances flexibility.

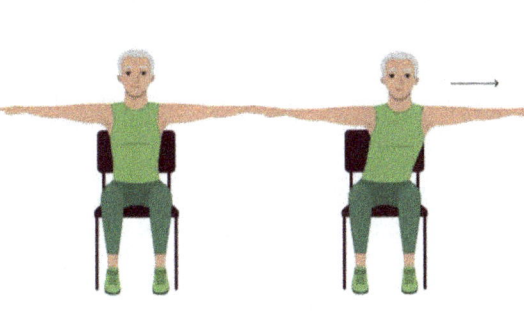

- Sit in the middle of a chair with your back unsupported
- Extend both arms straight to the sides at shoulder height or lower.
- Lean to one side, and avoid twisting.
- Return to center and repeat on the other side.
- Do 10-15 repetitions and 2-4 sets.

SEATED LUMBAR STABILIZATION: -Purpose -Focuses on stabilizing the lower back and strengthening the core to prevent lower back pain.

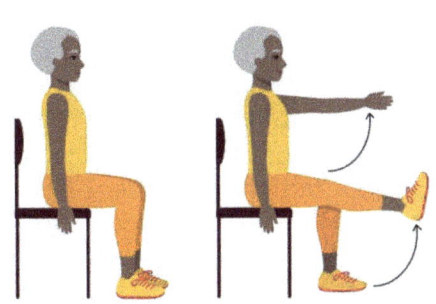

- Sit in the middle of your chair with your back straight and unsupported.
- Let your arms rest comfortably by your sides.
- Tighten your abdominal muscles, and while maintaining this tension, lift one foot slightly off the ground while raising the opposite arm over your head or to shoulder height.
- Hold for a count of 5, then alternate with the other foot and arm.
- Do 10-15 repetitions and 2-4 sets.

SEATED UPPER ABDOMINAL CRUNCHES: Purpose: -Strengthens the rectus abdominis, the muscles at the front of the abdomen; allows bending forward and helps core strength.
CAUTION: Do not do this exercise if you have spinal osteoporosis or compression fractures, a fused spine, or other conditions that require flexing at the waist, which is a contraindication. If you are unsure, please consult your physician before doing this exercise.

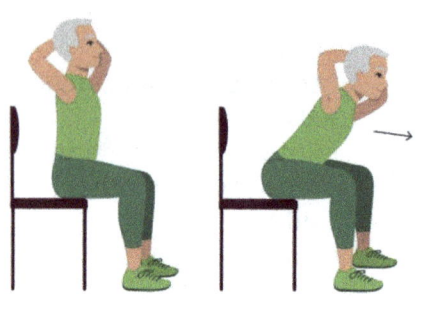

- Sit in the middle of a chair with your back unsupported
- Place your hands behind your head or cross them over your chest.
- Breathe in, and as you exhale, crunch forward by contracting your upper abdominal muscles, trying to bring your chest to your knees.
- As you inhale, return to the starting position.
- Do 10-15 repetitions and 2-4 sets.

SEATED LOWER ABDOMINAL CRUNCHES: Purpose: This exercise targets the lower portion of the abdomen, which is essential for pelvic stability and lower back support.

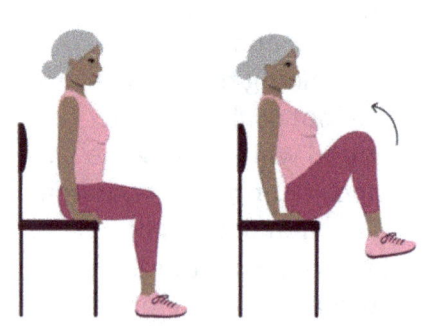

- Sit in the middle of a chair with your back unsupported
- Extend your legs slightly or keep them bent at the knees.
- Lean back and breathe in. As you exhale, lift your knees towards your chest.
- Inhale as you lower your legs, but don't let them touch the floor before going up again if you can.
- Do 10-15 repetitions and 2-4 sets.

Modification: - Do 1 leg at a time.

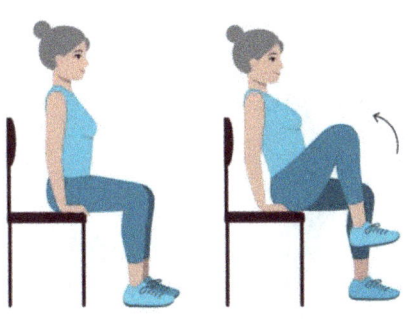

- Sit in the middle of a chair with your back unsupported
- Lean back to engage your core and breathe in. As you exhale, lift one knee toward your chest. Keep your back straight.
- Inhale as you lower your leg, but don't let it touch the floor before going up again if you can.
- Do 10-15 repetitions and 2-4 sets for each leg.

SEATED ABDOMINAL CRUNCH WITH A TWIST: Purpose -This targets the obliques, which are often less engaged in standard abdominal exercises but vital for lateral movement and spinal rotation.

CAUTION: Do not do this exercise if you have spinal osteoporosis or compression fractures, vertebral disc problems, a fused spine, or other conditions for which flexing at the waist is a contraindication. If you are unsure, please consult your physician.

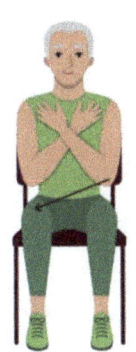 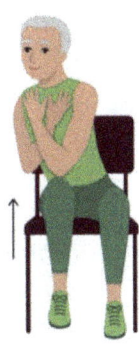

- Sit in the middle of a chair, with your back unsupported, and your arms crossed.
- Breathe in and as you exhale, bring one elbow toward the opposite knee while raising that knee to meet the elbow. (do not round your back
- Keep your head up.
- Inhale and return to the starting position.
- Repeat on the other side.
- Do 10-15 repetitions and 2-4 sets.

CHAIR PLANK: <u>Purpose</u>- Engages the entire core, promoting endurance and stability. Strengthens the abs, back, and shoulders..

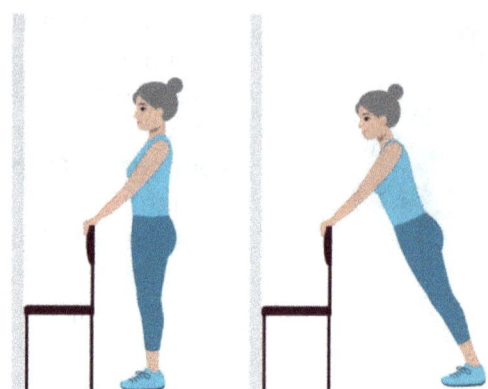

- Brace the chair against a sturdy object.
- Place your hands on the back of the chair with your elbows straight.
- Extend your legs back one at a time. Your body forms a straight line from your head to your heels.
- Hold for a count of 5, then return to standing.
- Perform five repetitions and do 2–4 sets.

Modification

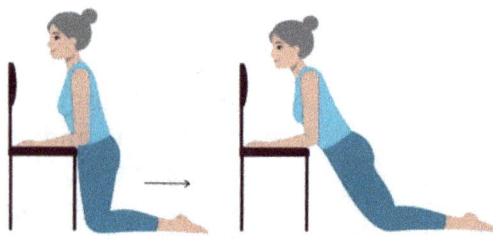

- Kneel in front of the chair, then place your forearms on the chair's seat, elbows directly under your shoulders.
- Extend your legs back one at a time. Your hips should be down, and your body forms a straight line from your head to your knees.
- Hold for a count of 5, then return to a relaxed position.
- Perform five repetitions and do 2–4 sets.

Progression:

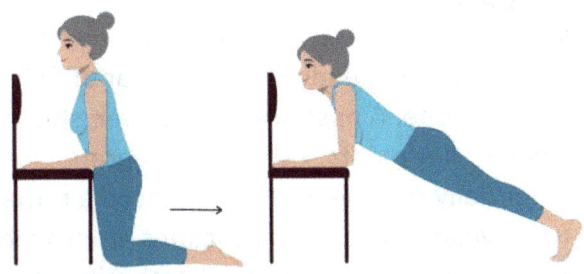

- Kneel in front of the chair, place your forearms on the chair's seat, and your elbows directly under your shoulders. Place a pad or pillow under your knees.
- Extend your legs back one at a time. Your hips should be down, and your body should form a straight line from your head to your heels.
- Hold for a count of 5, then return to a relaxed position.
- Perform five repetitions and do 2–4 sets.

Core strength isn't just about physical fitness; it's crucial for living independently and confidently. Incorporating these exercises into your daily routine will build strength and stability, making everyday activities easier and promoting an active, healthy lifestyle. Think of the chair as a tool and a partner in your journey, supporting you through movements that fortify your core and enrich your life. With regular practice, expect better balance, a lower risk of falls, and empowerment to seize each day's possibilities.

Chapter 5: Enhancing Balance through Exercise

Like a masterfully played violin, balance requires consistent practice to perform at its peak. Picture a woman who once avoided even the simplest of outings; her unsteady steps and fear of falling confined her to the safety of her home. A passionate gardener, she had relinquished the joy of tending to her plants. Yet, after integrating targeted balance exercises into her daily routine, she experienced a remarkable change. Her ability to navigate diverse landscapes improved dramatically, restoring her confidence to rejoin social gatherings and return to her beloved garden. This newfound stability underscores the transformative power of enhanced balance on one's quality of life.

Improved balance significantly enhances one's ability to move confidently and reduces the likelihood of falling. This aspect of physical health is crucial, particularly as one ages. The Centers for Disease Control and Prevention (CDC) reports that more than one in four Americans over the age of 65 experience a fall each year, making falls the leading cause of both fatal and nonfatal injuries among this demographic.

Falls can lead to serious consequences such as fractures, loss of independence, fear of further falls, and even long-term disability or death. Here's how dedicating time to balance training can be beneficial:

- <u>Prevention of Falls:</u> Balance exercises strengthen the muscles that keep you upright and enhance your body's coordination. Strong core and leg muscles can prevent or mitigate the risk of trips, slips, or stumbles.
- <u>Maintaining Independence:</u> By maintaining or improving your balance, you're more likely to continue performing daily activities without assistance, including simple tasks like walking to the mailbox, cooking, or bathing.
- <u>Confidence in Movement:</u> When you feel more stable, you'll likely engage more in physical and social activities. Confidence in your balance can lead to a more active lifestyle, supporting overall health.
- <u>Enhanced Life Quality:</u> Balance training can help you enjoy

simple pleasures, like walking in the park, dancing, or playing with grandchildren, without worrying about falling.

5.1 Balance and Fall Prevention Techniques

Offering exercise modifications is essential because balance capabilities vary among individuals. These adjustments cater to different fitness levels, ensuring everyone can participate safely and effectively. For those who require additional support, using a walker, cane, or countertop can provide the necessary stability during exercises. This support helps build confidence, allowing you to focus on the exercise without worrying about losing balance.

Additionally, adjusting your base of support can further tailor the exercise to your needs. A wider stance provides excellent stability, making the exercise easier. Conversely, a narrower stance can increase the challenge, offering a progression as your confidence and ability improve.

Regular practice plays a crucial role in improving balance. By setting a routine time for practice, you establish a habit that supports continuous improvement. Gradually increase the duration of your exercises as your stamina grows, ensuring that you challenge yourself while remaining within a safe and comfortable range. This gradual progression prevents overexertion, allowing you to build balance and coordination over time.

When performing standing exercises, engage your core muscles, which act as stabilizers, providing a solid foundation for balance. This engagement reduces the strain on your lower back and enhances the effectiveness of each exercise. Keep your shoulders relaxed and your back straight, allowing for proper alignment and reducing the risk of injury.

The following balance exercises are designed to be straightforward and safe, allowing you to practice them at home with minimal equipment.

Interactive Element: Balance Exercises

Consider using this checklist to help you incorporate balance exercises into your routine. By checking off each exercise as you complete it, you can monitor your progress and maintain motivation.

These exercises improve balance, coordination, and core strength, which are crucial for daily activities and fall prevention in seniors.

Perform these exercises with a sturdy chair or near a counter for immediate support (or use a walker or cane), and work within your comfort zone.

Once an exercise becomes easy, you can increase the number of repetitions and/or sets or add holding a weight to simulate activities of daily living. After mastering these balance exercises, you can challenge yourself even more by performing them using a standing pad or on the grass.

If using your chair, brace it against a wall or a counter so it does not move. Wear good-fitting, supportive shoes to prevent slipping. Most importantly, move within a pain-free range.

STANDING HEAD NOD AND TURN: <u>Purpose</u>- This exercise improves neck mobility and balance. Move your head slowly to prevent dizziness.

Head Nod

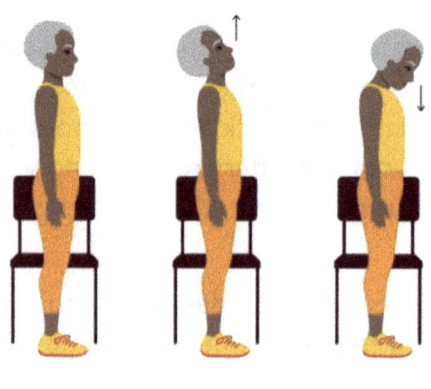

- Stand near a chair, countertop, or use a walker to place one or both hands on.
- Stand with your feet close together.
- Slowly look up, then down.
- Perform 10-15 repetitions. Do 2-4 sets.

Head Turn

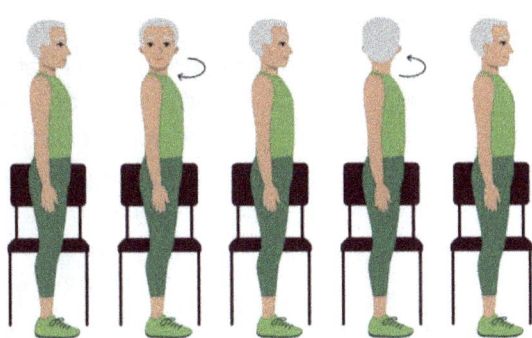

- Stand with your feet close together. Keep your arms relaxed by your sides.
- Slowly turn your head to look over one shoulder and back to the center.
- Then, slowly turn your head to look over the other shoulder and back to the center.
- Perform 10-15 repetitions. Do 2-4 sets.

Modification- Widen your stance. This broader base provides more stability, making it easier to maintain balance.

Progression

- Reduce the support to just one hand, then a finger or two, and then no hands.
- Narrow your base of support and bring your feet closer together.
- Close your eyes for short periods, which significantly challenges balance.
- Turn your head and shoulders to look behind you.

STANDING HEEL AND TOE RAISES: Purpose- Strengthens the calf and shin muscles to promote ankle range of motion balance

Heel Raises

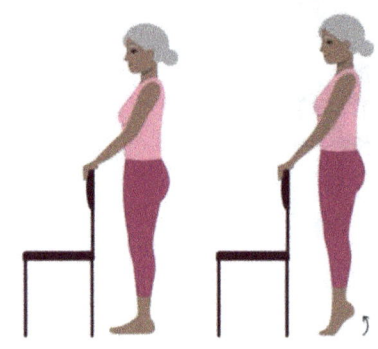

- Stand near a chair, countertop, or use a walker to place one or both hands on.
- Stand with your feet close together.
- Slowly lift your heels off the ground, rising onto your toes. Keep your body straight.
- Hold for a second or two, then lower your heels back to the ground slowly.
- Perform 10-15 repetitions. Do 2-4 sets.

Toe Raises

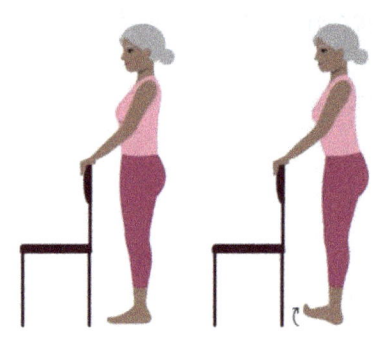

- Lift your toes off the ground, shifting your weight onto your heels. Your feet should form a "V" shape.
- Keep your knees straight but not locked.
- Hold for a second or two, then lower your heels back to the ground slowly.
- Perform 10-15 repetitions. Do 2-4 sets.

Modification- Widen your stance. This broader base provides more stability, making it easier to maintain balance.

Progression

- Reduce the support to just one hand, then a finger or two, then no hands.
- Narrow your base of support and bring your feet closer together.
- Close your eyes for short periods, which significantly challenges balance.

SINGLE LEG STANCE: Purpose- To enhance balance, strengthen the standing leg and core muscles.

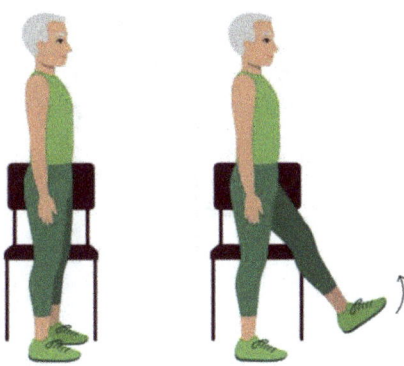

- Stand near a chair, countertop, or use a walker to place one or both hands on.
- Stand with your feet close together, then lift one leg off the ground.
- Bend the knee of the raised leg so the foot is behind you or extend it straight in front of you.
- Hold the leg out for 1-2 seconds, then lower it back down
- Keep your core engaged and do not lock the knee of the standing leg.
- Don't hold your breath; immediately lower the leg back to the ground if you feel unstable.
- Perform 10-15 repetitions. Do 2-4 sets.

Progression:

- Once you're comfortable, try reducing the support to just one hand, then a finger or two, and finally, no hands.
- Close your eyes for short periods.

STANDING SIDE LEG LIFT: Purpose- To strengthen the muscles on the side of the hip and improve lateral balance.

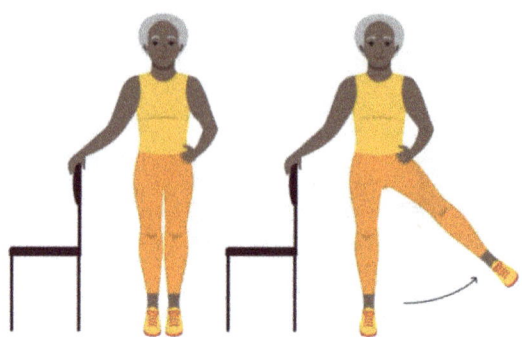

- Stand near a chair, countertop, or use a walker to place one or both hands on.
- Stand with your feet close together, then lift one leg off the ground to the side without leaning; about knee level is sufficient.
- Keep your hips and feet facing forward and hold the leg out for 1-2 seconds, then lower it back down
- Keep your core engaged and do not lock the knee of the standing leg.
- Don't hold your breath; immediately lower the leg back to the ground if you feel unstable.
- Perform 10-15 repetitions. Do 2-4 sets.

Progression

- Once you're comfortable, try reducing the support to just one hand, then a finger or two, and finally, no hands.
- Add ankle weights for increased resistance, but only if your balance is secure.
- Close your eyes for short periods.

SIDESTEPPING AND GRAPEVINE: <u>Purpose</u>- To work on coordination, balance, leg strength, and hip mobility.

Basic Side Stepping:

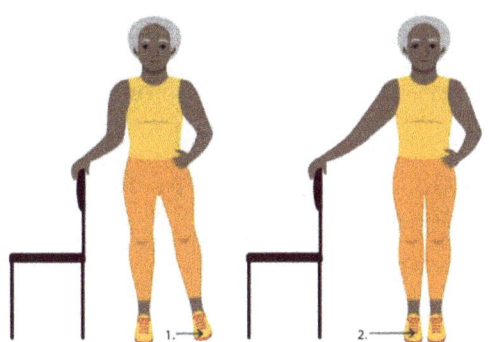

- ○ Stand near a chair, countertop, or use a walker to place one or both hands on.
- ○ Start with your feet together and step to the side with one foot (e.g., your right foot).
- ○ Keep your toes and hips facing forward, not diagonally or to the side, then bring the left foot next to the right foot, but not passing it.
- ○ Perform 10-15 steps, and do 2-4 sets in each direction.

Grapevine Variation:

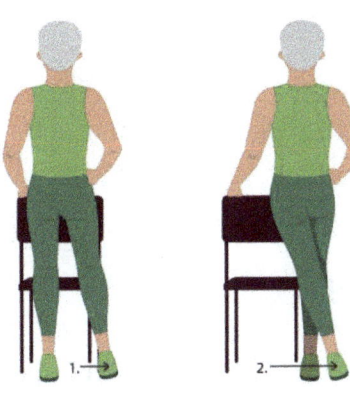

- ○ Step to the side with your right foot.
- ○ Cross your left foot behind your right foot.
- ○ Step to the right again with your right foot.
- ○ Cross your left foot in front of your right foot.
- ○ Step to the right again with your right foot.
- ○ Continue this pattern for a few steps, then reverse to move in the other direction.
- ○ Perform 10-15 steps, and do 2-4 sets in each direction.

Progression:

- Once you're comfortable, try reducing the support on the counter with just one hand, then a finger or two, then no hands.
- Increase the width of your steps.
- Increase the speed of your side steps.
- Try closing your eyes for a few steps to heighten the balance challenge.

FORWARD STEP OR TANDEM STEP: <u>Purpose</u> - This exercise enhances core strength and improves balance and stability. Perform 3-5 times each leg, and do 2-4 sets.

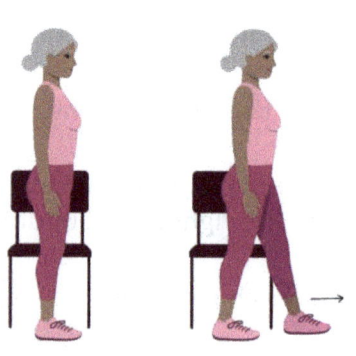

- Stand near a chair, countertop, or use a walker to place one or both hands on.
- Stand with your feet as close together as comfortably. Then, step one foot forward.
- Keep your arms at your sides or extend them to the sides. Look straight ahead.
- Hold this position for 10 to 30 seconds, then step back and repeat on the other foot.

Progression:

- Once you're comfortable, try reducing the support on the counter with just one hand, then a finger or two, then no hands.
- Increase the width of your steps.
- Reduce your base of support and bring your feet closer together until you can stand in tandem.
- Slowly look from one side to another and up and down.
- Close your eyes for a few seconds.

STANDING REACHING: Purpose- To improve core strength and overall balance for reaching activities.

Side Reach:

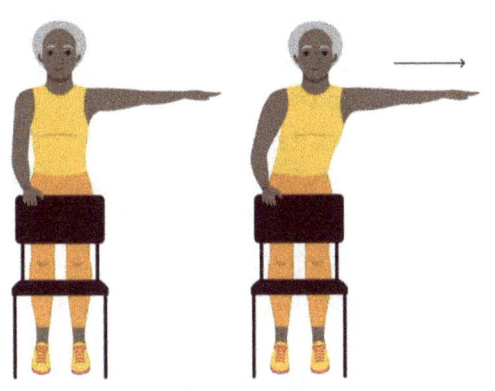

- ◦ Stand with feet shoulder-width apart, facing the support.
- ◦ With one hand on the support, extend the other arm at shoulder height, reaching to the side.
- ◦ The movement should come from the trunk, not the whole body leaning.
- ◦ Perform 10-15 in each direction, and do 2-4 sets.

Forward Reach:

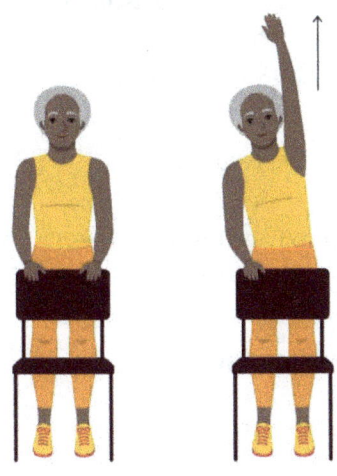

- ◦ Stand with feet shoulder-width apart, facing the support.
- ◦ With one hand on the support, extend the other arm upward, reaching as high as possible, as if grabbing something from a high shelf.
- ◦ Perform 10-15 in each direction, and do 2-4 sets.

Diagonal Reach:

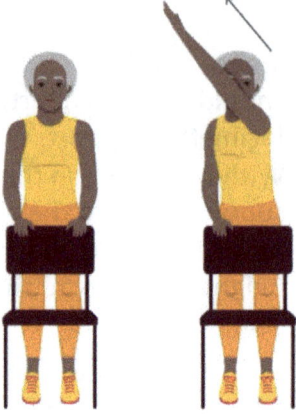

- Stand with feet shoulder-width apart, facing the support.
- With one hand on the support, reach the opposite arm diagonally across your body, as high and far as is comfortable, keeping your hips forward.
- Perform 10-20 in each direction, and do 2-4 sets.

Progression:

- Once you're comfortable, try reducing the support on the counter with just a finger or two, then no hands.
- Place your feet closer together, narrowing your base of support.
- Increase the stretch or the height of the reach as flexibility and balance improve.
- Gently rotate your torso toward the extended arm, then return to the center. This adds a rotational core component.
- Lift one leg slightly off the ground while reaching.

BOX STEP and WALTZ STEP: <u>Purpose-</u> To enhance dynamic balance, coordination, and leg strength by practicing a basic stepping pattern like in ballroom dancing. Stand near a chair, countertop, or use a walker to place one or both hands on. Holding a cane provides additional support.

Box Step

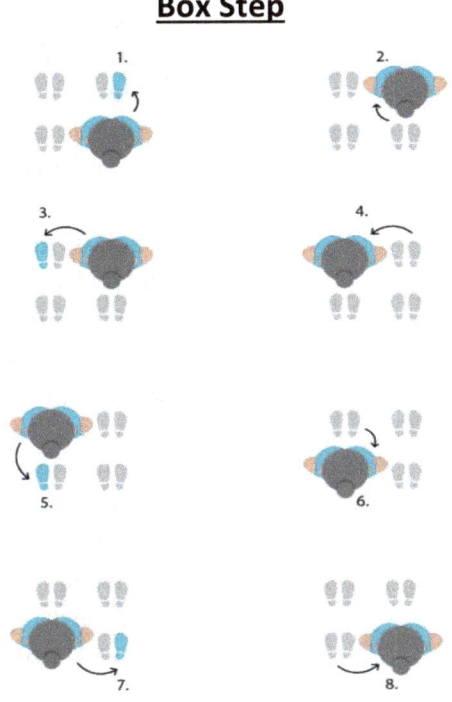

- **Forward Step**: Step forward with your right foot.
- Bring your left foot forward to meet your right, closing the step. You should have both feet together again.
- **Side Step Left**: Step to the side with your left foot.
- Bring your right foot over to meet your left foot, closing the step again.
- **Backward Step**: Step back with your left foot.
- Bring your right foot back to meet your left foot, closing the step. You should have both feet together again.
- **Side Step Right**: Step to the side with your right foot.
- Bring your left foot over to meet your right foot, close the step again, and return to your original position.
- Maintain an upright posture, looking slightly ahead to aid balance.

Waltz Step

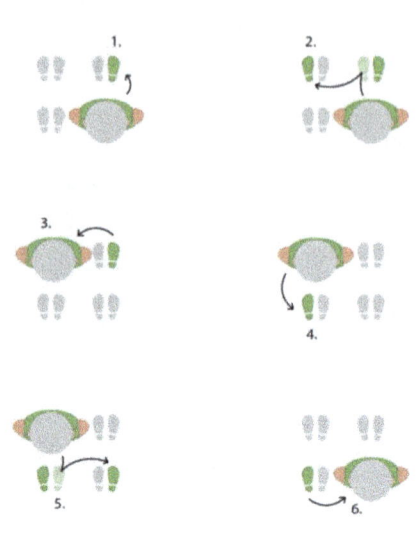

- ○ **Forward Step**: Step forward with your right foot.
- ○ Bring your left foot forward, not placing it on the ground. Instead, swing it forward and to the left side, then put your foot on the ground and bring your right foot over to meet it (like in a waltz dance step).
- ○ **Backward Step**: Step back with your left foot.
- ○ Bring your right foot back; do not place it on the ground; instead, swing it back and to the right, then put it on the ground, and bring your left foot over to meet it.
- ○ This will complete the box and return you to your original position.

Progression:

- ○ As balance improves, reduce the support by using fewer fingers or just the fingertips on the chair or counter, eventually trying to perform the steps with minimal or no support.
- ○ Increase the step length slightly or add a gentle sway or arm movement to mimic dance-like movements.
- ○ Switch the lead foot and go in the other direction.
- ○ Add music with a slow beat to help with the timing and enjoyment of the movement.

Balance exercises are not just about preventing falls; they empower you to live fully and confidently. Integrating these practices into your routine enhances your ability to participate in the activities you love, navigate your environment quickly, and maintain independence.

> *"The best way to find yourself is to lose yourself in the service of others." - Mahatma Gandhi.*

People who give without expecting anything in return live happier lives. So, let's work together to make a difference!

Would you help someone like you who is curious about "Chair Yoga Revolution for Seniors" but unsure where to start?

My mission is to make chair exercises accessible, easy, and fun for everyone. But to reach more people, I need your help.

Most folks pick books based on what others say about them. So, I'm asking you to help another senior by leaving a review.

It costs nothing and takes less than a minute, but it could change someone's life. Your review could help:

- One more family member helps their loved one.
- One more small business supports the senior community.
- One more senior do something they love
- One more person get stronger and healthier
- One more dream come true.

To make a difference, leave a review:

If you love helping others, you're my kind of person. Thank you from the bottom of my heart!

S. Carroll, MPT

Chapter 6: Cardiovascular Focus

In my years as a physical therapist, I encountered many patients with cardiac problems who required rehabilitation. One encounter remains particularly vivid. I met a gentleman in his late 60s who underwent cardiac catheterization to improve the blood flow to his heart. This gentleman was sedentary, seriously overweight, and had arthritis in his knees, which made walking difficult. His cardiologist was adamant that he begin exercising 15 minutes to 30 minutes a day. The gentleman could not walk from his bedroom to his kitchen without experiencing severe shortness of breath or pain in his knees. He was discouraged and did not believe he could follow his cardiologist's instructions. I introduced him to chair yoga exercises and convinced him that by starting a slow and consistent routine, gradually increasing the duration, and adding resistance, he could exercise for 15 to 30 minutes daily within four to six weeks. This gentleman found that he could efficiently perform the chair yoga program designed for him, which gave him the confidence to be consistent with the program, as it did not increase his knee pain. He could increase the intensity of the exercises in the seated position without becoming too short of breath. After a couple of weeks of chair yoga, he could incorporate simple standing exercises. A couple of weeks later, with the aid of a cane, he began a walking program to supplement his chair yoga exercise routine.

6.1 Using a Chair for Cardiovascular Exercise

Specific chair yoga sequences can enhance cardiovascular benefits. For instance, chair aerobics and chair boxing are excellent for elevating the heart rate and promoting cardiovascular endurance. This exercise involves raising and lowering the arms and legs in various patterns, engaging the upper and lower body in a coordinated effort. Such exercises increase heart rate in a controlled manner, similar to brisk walking or cycling, yet they remain gentle enough to accommodate individuals of varying fitness levels. Chair cardio exercises are low-impact, making them ideal for those who find standing exercises challenging. They help maintain circulation, which is especially beneficial for those who spend long periods stationary due to health or mobility constraints.

The beauty of chair exercises is their adaptability. You can adjust the pace to match your fitness level, ensuring everyone can participate without strain.

Over time, each sequence of chair-based exercises can do the following.

- Strengthen the Heart: These exercises can help the heart work more efficiently to pump blood.
- Boost Endurance: Regular practice increases the duration of physical activity without tiring.
- Improve Circulation: Moving the limbs helps prevent blood stagnation and supports better oxygenation of muscles and organs.
- Aid in Weight Management: Increased heart rate and metabolism help burn calories, even at a lower intensity than traditional aerobic exercises.

Incorporating cardio chair yoga sequences into a daily routine can be a game-changer for those seeking to maintain or improve their cardiovascular health in a way that's accessible, enjoyable, and suitable for all fitness levels. It's a testament to how even small, controlled movements can yield significant health benefits if done consistently.

Personal Reflection: Setting Your Heart Health Goals

Take a moment to reflect on your journey to heart health. What are your current cardiovascular goals, and how do you envision chair yoga helping you achieve them? Consider setting small, attainable goals to track your progress over time. For example, you may aim to maintain stable blood pressure, reduce shortness of breath with activity, lose weight, or reduce medication dependency. Grab a piece of paper or a logbook, jot down your intentions, and revisit them as you progress through this book, adjusting as needed to reflect your evolving health journey.

With dedication and consistency, chair yoga can offer a gentle yet effective path to a healthier heart, much like it has done for hundreds of seniors.

Interactive Element: Cardiovascular Exercises

Any exercise routine will elevate your heart rate, providing cardiovascular exercise. If you want to incorporate a cardiovascular component into your exercise routine and further elevate your heart rate, consider the following.

Use low or no weight as a starting point and perform these exercises quickly (at least once every second). Sustain the movement as long as possible, aiming for between 30 and 60 seconds, and do 3 to 5 repetitions.

CHAIR AEROBICS: Purpose- Combines upper and lower body movements to elevate the heart rate, improving cardiovascular endurance and coordination. It also engages core muscles for stability.

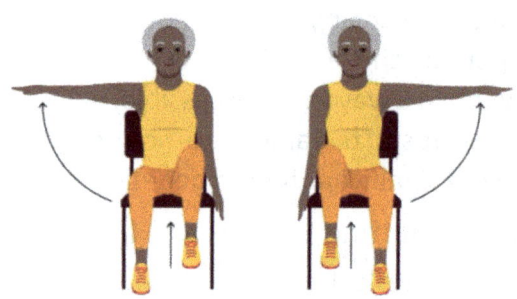

- ○ Sit at the edge of your chair with your feet firmly on the ground, your back straight, and your hands resting at your sides.
- ○ Alternate raising your right arm to the side to shoulder height while lifting your left knee towards your chest, then switch to the left arm and right knee.
- ○ Keep this movement brisk but controlled, aiming for coordination between arm and leg movements.

SEATED JUMPING JACKS: <u>Purpose</u>- Simulates standing jumping jacks for cardiovascular challenge while seated, promoting coordination, and increased heart rate.

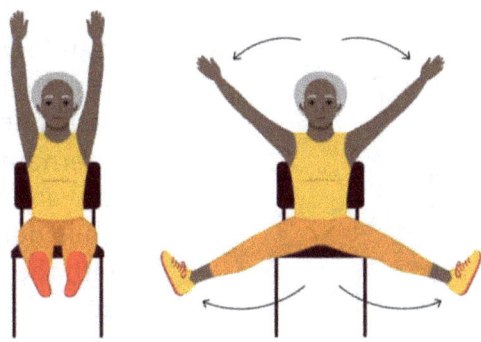

- Sit at the edge of your chair with your feet on the ground and your hands resting at your side.
- Lift your legs, spread them apart, then bring them back together and place your feet back on the ground. Simultaneously, raise your arms out to the side and over your head, mimicking a jumping jack.
- Return to the starting position and repeat at a quick pace.

Modification: Do one side at a time, lifting one leg and arm together on one side (half of a jumping jack), then switch sides.

CHAIR RUNNING: Purpose: Elevates the heart rate, providing a seated workout for the legs, core, and arms.

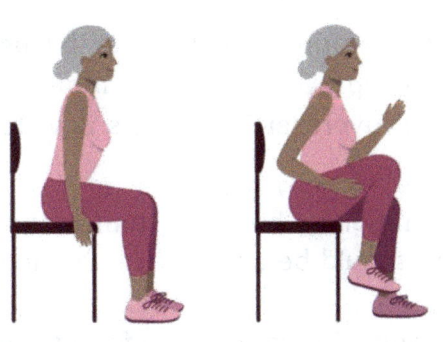

- Lean forward slightly in your chair.
- Begin by lifting your knees alternately as if you're jogging in place.
- Hold your arms at your sides with your elbows bent, and move them in time with your knees, simulating a running motion.
- Keep the movements quick and rhythmic.

PUNCH AND KICK COMBO: Purpose- Elevates heart rate, improves coordination, and engages multiple muscle groups, providing a dynamic form of seated cardio.

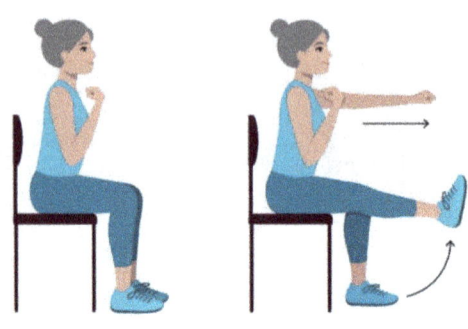

- Lean forward slightly in your chair, or rest your back if needed.
- Alternate punching forward with each arm while doing small kicks with the opposite leg. For example, punch with your right arm as you kick with your left leg, then switch.
- Keep the movements controlled but as fast as comfortably possible.

WALKING OR BIKING PROGRAM

Adding a walking or stationary bike program is a great way to kickstart cardiovascular fitness. Start small - aim for a few days a week to begin with. Wear comfortable, supportive shoes to protect your feet and joints. If you need support while walking due to balance or mobility issues, a walker or cane can help reduce energy expenditure, maintain safety and comfort, and allow you to walk further and longer.

Following these steps when incorporating a walking or biking program into your exercise routine will improve cardiovascular health and minimize symptoms of overuse or overexertion. Here's how to begin:

- Time yourself walking or riding a stationary bike at a comfortable pace for as long as possible. You should be able to breathe and converse easily.
- Stop when you become tired or short of breath, and refrain from pushing yourself further. For example, if you manage five minutes, that's your starting point.

- Maintain this activity at the determined pace and time for at least a week (or possibly two) before increasing the time or the pace.
- Listen to your body. If you experience pain or fatigue, stop immediately.
- When you're ready, test yourself again by timing how long you can go before needing to stop or rest. Don't be surprised if you only add one or two minutes; this is normal and shows progress.
- Set this new duration as your baseline for another week or two before you try to increase your time or speed again.

Chapter 7: Adapting Chair Yoga for Limited Mobility

The concept of chair yoga and exercise modification is not merely about adjusting poses; it's about fostering an inclusive environment where everyone, regardless of their physical limitations, can participate and benefit. This philosophy is particularly significant for seniors who may experience a limited range of motion or endurance. Personalized exercise routines acknowledge these unique needs, offering adaptations that make yoga accessible. By modifying exercises, we create opportunities for participation that might otherwise be unattainable, allowing individuals to engage at their comfort level.

One of the most effective ways to adapt common chair yoga poses is through specific modifications that accommodate limited movement. For instance, using pillows for added support can significantly enhance comfort during seated exercises. Placing a pillow behind the back or under the hips can provide additional cushioning, reducing strain and promoting proper alignment. Similarly, reducing the depth of seated forward bends allows those with limited flexibility to participate without overexertion. By bending only as far as feels comfortable, individuals can enjoy the benefits of the exercise without risking injury. Additionally, slightly or significantly bending the elbow and knee joints can minimize strain and torque on the joints while still engaging the muscles. These modifications ensure that the exercises remain safe and effective, regardless of one's physical condition.

Props can facilitate modifications, helping to achieve correct form and enhancing comfort during yoga practice. Yoga blocks can be invaluable for those who need extra reach or support. Sturdy household items, such as thick books, can serve as adequate substitutes if yoga blocks are unavailable. These props can be placed under the hands or feet during seated poses, providing stability and allowing individuals to maintain proper alignment. Straps, too, are essential tools for extending reach and deepening stretches. Using a strap allows one to hold a pose more comfortably, ensuring the stretch is both safe and beneficial. These tools empower individuals to engage fully in their practice, adapting each pose to their unique needs.

Listening to your body is crucial for a safe and effective yoga practice. Recognizing personal limits and adapting exercises is essential to avoid discomfort and pain. Progression in exercising should be gradual, allowing your body to adjust and strengthen over time. You can increase the repetitions, weight, or duration as your endurance and strength improve with each exercise. It's essential to remember that exercising is not about pushing beyond your capabilities, but about nurturing both your body and mind. If a pose feels uncomfortable or causes pain, it's a signal to modify the exercise or take a break.

7.1 Using Support for Safe Standing Exercises

Standing exercises can seem daunting for many seniors, especially those concerned about maintaining their balance. However, using the back of your chair, a cane, a walker, or a counter as a supportive tool can make these exercises safer and more accessible. A cane or walker, typically viewed as just a mobility aid, can be a reliable partner in your exercise routine. Its stability offers reassurance, enabling you to perform standing poses with confidence. You can maintain an upright position by holding an assistive device while focusing on the exercises. This support is crucial for movements that involve shifting weight or balance, reducing the risk of falls, and enhancing safety during practice.

Using assistive devices in your standing exercises fosters independence and empowerment, allowing you to try movements that might otherwise seem challenging. As you exercise regularly, your core and lower body strength will improve, potentially lessening your reliance on those devices.

Chapter 8 Using Progress Logs for Motivation

Many seniors express frustration with what they describe as the "invisible treadmill"—the sensation of working hard but not seeing any progress. They might begin a new fitness regimen, only to feel disheartened when they don't notice immediate, tangible results. Here's where the magic of keeping a progress log comes in. By recording their activities, seniors can track their accomplishments and observe the subtle yet significant gains in strength, balance, and endurance. Each entry in their log is a testament to their perseverance, turning what feels like abstract effort into concrete achievements. This chapter examines how such documentation can serve as a powerful motivator, particularly when progress appears to be out of sight.

8.1 The Benefits of Tracking Progress

Tracking progress is more than just a method for monitoring changes; it's a powerful motivator that can sustain your enthusiasm and commitment over time. By keeping a record of your achievements, you allow yourself to reflect on your growth, providing tangible evidence of your hard work and dedication. This practice can help transform exercise from a daunting task into an empowering experience. This visual representation of success can be the encouragement you need on days when motivation wanes.

Setting small, achievable goals is a cornerstone of effective progress tracking. These goals serve as stepping stones, guiding you toward more significant accomplishments. By breaking down larger objectives into manageable tasks, you create a clear roadmap that leads to your desired outcomes. This method makes the process more approachable and allows for frequent celebrations of success, which are crucial for maintaining motivation.

Celebrating milestones and improvements is an integral part of the progress-tracking process. Recognizing these moments of success acknowledges your hard work and reminds you of the positive changes you are experiencing. Acknowledging progress creates a positive feedback loop, reinforcing the connection between effort and outcome.

In addition to personal celebrations, consider finding ways to share your achievements with others. Engaging with a supportive community, whether it's family, friends, or fellow exercise enthusiasts, can amplify the joy of success. Sharing your progress with others fosters a sense of camaraderie and accountability, motivating you to stay committed to your routine. This social aspect of progress tracking can also inspire others to pursue their own goals, creating a ripple effect of positivity and encouragement. By participating in a community, you gain access to a network of support that can help you navigate challenges and celebrate victories together.

8.2 Establish a Realistic Timeline for Improvement

Starting a new exercise routine can raise the question of when to anticipate results. Setting a realistic timeline that aligns with your goals and current fitness level is crucial. Generally, if you're consistent with your workouts, you can expect to see improvements in balance, strength, and endurance within four to six weeks.

This period allows your body to adjust to new activities, enhancing muscle memory and strength. However, if you're not sticking to a regular schedule, it may take longer than six weeks to see changes. Recognizing this variability is key to managing expectations and avoiding disappointment.

Understanding the physiological changes that occur during this period can provide valuable insight into the process. Initially, your body undergoes neuromuscular adaptations, allowing the nervous system to communicate more efficiently with your muscles. This communication improves coordination and balance, even before significant muscle growth is evident. As you exercise regularly, your muscles strengthen, enhancing your endurance and ability to perform daily activities more efficiently. These changes are gradual, often imperceptible on a daily basis, but they accumulate over time, resulting in measurable improvements in your physical capabilities.

A progress log is valuable for tracking your achievements over time, whether by maintaining a detailed record of activities or keeping a journal with daily or weekly entries that focus on exercises. This documentation provides a comprehensive overview of your journey, highlighting challenges and triumphs. It also allows you to see tangible progress, like when an exercise becomes easier, signaling increased strength or improved endurance. It offers opportunities for reflection, enabling the identification of patterns, evaluation of progress, and informed adjustments to your routine. Thus, it supports continuous improvement and alignment with your goals.

When considering how to progress your exercises, it's essential to focus on three key aspects: resistance, sets, and repetitions. These elements can be adjusted incrementally to ensure continued results and avoid plateaus. An effective method for progression is to change the number of sets and repetitions. As you become more comfortable with a particular exercise, consider increasing the number of repetitions by 5-10 or adding an extra set to your routine. This incremental increase enhances endurance and muscle stamina, enabling you to perform exercises for longer periods without fatigue. However, balancing these increments with adequate rest and recovery is essential to prevent overuse injuries and ensure sustainable progress.

Next, increase resistance by adding weight or using more challenging exercise variations. For example, if you have been using water bottles for arm exercises, consider gradually increasing your weight or switching to heavier household items. This increase in resistance challenges your muscles further, promoting additional strength gains.

Do not increase the reps, sets, or weights you lift until you consistently perform your exercise routine for at least 5-7 days. If your workout schedule is three days a week, wait two to three weeks before making any increases. This schedule will allow your body time to adapt to the new exercises, reducing the risk of overuse injuries such as pain or inflammation by avoiding excessive stress on your muscles and tendons.

Incorporating these strategies into your exercise routine supports ongoing development and fosters a sense of accomplishment and motivation. As you continue to engage with your logs, you'll find that they become more than just a record of activities—they become a source of inspiration, guiding you toward new achievements and possibilities.

Reflection Section: Designing Your Exercise and Progress Plan

Designing a progress plan tailored to your unique needs and goals is essential to your fitness journey. Use the following questions to guide your reflection and planning:

- What improvements do you hope to achieve in your balance, strength, or endurance?
- How often can you realistically commit to exercising each week?
- What exercises have you enjoyed or found beneficial, and how can you incorporate them?
- Are there particular areas where you feel challenged, and how might you address these in your plan?
- How will you track your progress, and what will you do to celebrate milestones along the way?

Reflecting on these questions can help you create a personalized plan that aligns with your goals and lifestyle.

SAMPLE ROUTINES TO CONSIDER

Here are some suggestions for weekly exercise routines incorporating strengthening and balance elements. Remember to include at least one rest day in your week.

Start with less resistance than you think you can handle, or no resistance at all, to prevent overstressing your tendons and muscles. Once the exercise becomes easy, you can increase the number of repetitions and/or sets or add weight. Most importantly, move your joints within a pain-free range. Remember to practice breathing techniques. It is also a good idea to incorporate one cardio exercise into your daily routine.

3 DAY ROUTINE

DAY 1
- 4 Arm Exercises - Overhead Press, Biceps Curl, Lateral Arm Raises, Front Arm Raises
- 4 Leg Exercises - Seated Marching, Seated Kicks, Inner Thigh Squeeze, Heel Raises
- 4 Core Exercises - Seated Torso Twist, Seated Leaning Front and Back, Chair Plank, Seated Lower Abdominal Crunches
- 4 Balance Exercises - Standing Head Nod and Turn, Standing Heel and Toe Raises, Side Stepping or Grapevine, Single Leg Stance
- 1 Cardio Exercise of your choosing
- Stretching Exercises

DAY 2
- 4 Balance Exercises - Standing Leg Side Lift, Standing Head Nod and Turn, Box Step, Side Stepping, or Grapevine
- 4 Core Exercises - Seated Abdominal Crunch with a Twist, Seated Torso Twist, Seated Lumbar Stabilization, Seated Leaning Front and Back
- 1 Cardio Exercise of your choosing
- Stretching Exercises

DAY 3
- 4 Arm Exercises - Shoulder and Triceps Extension, Seated Chair Press, Wrist and Forearm Strengthening, Chest Opener
- 4 Leg Exercises- Seated Leg Lift, Chair Squat, Toe Raises, Leg Open/Close
- 4 Core Exercises - Seated Upper Abdominal Crunch, Seated Abdominal Crunch with a Twist, Seated Lumbar Stabilization, Seated Side Reaching
- 4 Balance Exercises - Standing Side Leg Lift, Forward Step or Tandem Step, Box Step, Standing Reach
- 1 Cardio Exercise of Your Choosing
- Stretching Exercises

4 DAY ROUTINE

DAY 1 AND 3

- 4 Arm Exercises - Overhead Press, Biceps Curl, Lateral Arm Raises, Front Arm Raises
- 4 Leg Exercises - Seated Marching, Seated Kicks, Inner Thigh Squeeze, Heel Raises
- 4 Core Exercises - Seated Torso Twist, Seated Leaning Front and Back, Chair Plank, Seated Lower Abdominal Crunches
- 4 Balance Exercises - Standing Head Nod and Turn, Standing Heel and Toe Raises, Side Stepping or Grapevine, Single Leg Stance
- 1 Cardio Exercise of your choosing
- Stretching Exercises

DAY 2 AND 4

- 4 Arm Exercises - Shoulder and Triceps Extension, Seated Chair Press, Wrist and Forearm Strengthening, Chest Opener
- 4 Leg Exercises- Seated Leg Lift, Chair Squat, Toe Raises, Leg Open/Close
- 4 Core Exercises - Seated Upper Abdominal Crunch, Seated Abdominal Crunch with a Twist, Seated Lumbar Stabilization, Seated Side Reaching
- 4 Balance Exercises - Standing Side Leg Lift, Forward Step or Tandem Step, Box Step, Standing Reach
- 1 Cardio Exercise of your choosing
- Stretching Exercises

5 DAY ROUTINE

DAY 1 AND 3

- 4 Arm Exercises - Overhead Press, Bicep Curl, Lateral Arm Raises, Front Arm Raises
- 4 Leg Exercises - Seated Marching, Seated Kicks, Inner Thigh Squeeze, Heel Raises
- 4 Core Exercises - Seated Torso Twist, Seated Leaning Front and Back, Chair Plank, Seated Lower Abdominal Crunches

- 4 Balance Exercises - Standing Head Nod and Turn, Standing Heel and Toe Raises, Side Stepping or Grapevine, Single Leg Stance
- 1 Cardio Exercise of your choosing
- Stretching Exercises

DAY 2 AND 4

- 4 Arm Exercises - Shoulder and Triceps Extension, Seated Chair Press, Wrist and Forearm Strengthening, Chest Opener
- 4 Leg Exercises- Seated Leg Lift, Chair Squat, Toe Raises, Leg Open/Close
- 4 Core Exercises - Seated Upper Abdominal Crunch, Seated Abdominal Crunch with a Twist, Seated Lumbar Stabilization, Seated Side Reaching
- 4 Balance Exercises - Standing Side Leg Lift, Forward Step or Tandem Step, Box Step, Standing Reach
- 1 Cardio Exercise of your choosing
- Stretching Exercises

DAY 5

- 2 Arm Exercises - Seated Chair Press, Bicep Curl
- 2 Leg Exercises - Chair Squat, Inner Thigh Squeeze
- 2 Core Exercises - Seated Abdominal Crunch with a Twist, Seated Leaning Front and Back
- 2 Balance Exercises - Forward Step or Tandem Step, Side Stepping or Grapevine
- 1 Cardio Exercise of your choosing
- Stretching Exercises

6 DAY ROUTINE

DAY 1, 3, AND 5

- 3 Arm Exercises - Overhead Press, Lateral Arm Raises, Front Arm Raises
- 3 Leg Exercises - Seated Marching, Seated Kicks, Heel Raises
- 3 Core Exercises - Seated Torso Twist, Chair Plank, Seated Lower Abdominal Crunches
- 3 Balance Exercises - Standing Head Nod and Turn, Standing

Heel and Toe Raises, Single Leg Stance
- 1 Cardio Exercise of your choosing
- Stretching Exercises

DAY 2 AND 4

- 3 Arm Exercises - Shoulder and Triceps Extension, Wrist and Forearm Strengthening, Chest Opener
- 3 Leg Exercises- Seated Leg Lift, Toe Raises, Leg Open/Close
- 3 Core Exercises - Seated Upper Abdominal Crunch, Seated Lumbar Stabilization, Seated Side Reaching
- 3 Balance Exercises - Standing Side Leg Lift, Box Step, Standing Reach
- 1 Cardio Exercise of your choosing
- Stretching Exercises

DAY 6

- 2 Arm Exercises - Seated Chair Press, Bicep Curl
- 2 Leg Exercises - Chair Squat, Inner Thigh Squeeze
- 2 Core Exercises - Seated Abdominal Crunch with a Twist, Seated Leaning Front and Back
- 2 Balance Exercises -Forward Step or Tandem Step, Side Stepping or Grapevine
- 1 Cardio Exercise of your choosing
- Stretching Exercises

As we conclude this chapter, it's clear that creating a weekly exercise routine and tracking progress is an invaluable tool in your exercise journey. Setting achievable goals and celebrating milestones builds a sense of accomplishment that fuels your commitment. The next chapter will explore the importance of flexibility and stretching in maintaining mobility and preventing injuries, thereby enhancing your overall exercise experience.

Chapter 9: Gentle Stretching for Joint, Muscle, and Mental Health

Imagine waking up with less stiffness that greets you each day. Improved flexibility is an achievable reality. The art of gentle stretching can transform your mornings into scenes of lightness and agility. Stretching is crucial in managing pain associated with joint conditions, and it is a natural and effective way to alleviate discomfort.

Regular stretching can be transformative for those managing arthritis or muscle stiffness. It can alleviate symptoms by improving the flexibility of the muscles and connective tissues.

Have you ever woken up feeling stiff and immobile? That's often due to prolonged inactivity overnight. Gentle stretching can be your morning hero. It counteracts stiffness by warming up your muscles and joints, enhancing flexibility and range of motion.

Incorporating regular stretching into your daily life enhances physical flexibility and offers psychological benefits that can significantly improve your mental well-being. The practice of mindful movement during stretching reduces stress by shifting focus away from daily worries, creating a meditative state that calms the mind. As you engage in these deliberate movements, your body releases tension, leading to a noticeable improvement in mood and energy levels. Stretching increases blood circulation, delivering vital oxygen and nutrients to your muscles and promoting a sense of vitality and alertness. By consistently stretching, you cultivate a routine that nurtures body and mind, fostering a holistic approach to health.

9.1 Holistic Benefits of Stretching

Stretching is particularly important for seniors due to several physiological changes that occur with age. Here are some essential points on why stretching is crucial for older adults:

<u>Maintenance of Muscle Flexibility and Joint Range of Motion</u>: As people age, muscles lose elasticity, and joints can become stiff, reducing their range of motion. Regular stretching can counteract these effects by keeping muscles flexible, strong, and healthy, which helps ease the performance of daily activities.

Prevention of Muscle Strain: Flexible muscles are less prone to injuries from sudden movements or falls, which can be more common in older adults.

Improvement in Balance and Coordination: Stretching improves balance, coordination, and postural alignment. Maintaining good balance is vital for seniors to prevent falls, a leading cause of injury in this population. Stretching can enhance proprioceptive feedback, which is the body's ability to sense its position in space, further aiding in better coordination.

Pain Management: Many seniors suffer from arthritis, a condition that causes the joints to become inflamed and painful. Gentle stretching can help alleviate joint pain and stiffness by enhancing circulation and reducing tension in the surrounding joints. Stretching the muscles around the spine can help alleviate back pain, a common complaint among older people, by supporting better posture and reducing muscle tightness.

Enhancement of Blood Circulation: Stretching the muscles of the lower extremities, including the calves, hamstrings, and quadriceps, can significantly enhance circulation, countering the effects of gravity on the legs. Stretching reduces muscle tension, which can otherwise compress blood vessels and restrict blood flow. Additionally, it helps maintain or improve the elasticity of veins, aiding in effective venous return and reducing swelling in the lower legs. This improved circulation also ensures that more oxygen and nutrients are delivered to the muscles, aiding in healing, reducing fatigue, and supporting overall muscle health, which is particularly beneficial for maintaining circulatory health in older adults.

Mental Health and Stress Reduction: Stretching can also serve as a meditative practice, helping to reduce stress and anxiety, which can benefit mental health, especially in seniors who may face increased anxiety about health or independence. Stretching releases endorphins, which are natural mood lifters, combating depression, which can be prevalent in older age groups.

Preparation for Other Physical Activities and Enhanced Performance: Stretching beforehand can help prepare muscles, reduce the risk of injury, and improve performance in activities such as walking, swimming, or gentle aerobics for seniors engaging in any form of exercise or physical therapy.

In summary, stretching is not just about maintaining physical health; it's integral to enhancing the quality of life, supporting independence, and promoting well-being in later years.

9.2 Range of Motion for Improved Mobility and Safety

Maintaining flexibility in your hips and knees is crucial for preserving mobility and independence. These joints bear a significant portion of the body's weight and play a pivotal role in daily activities, such as walking, bending, and standing. Simple tasks can become challenging without adequate flexibility, which can impact your ability to move freely and comfortably. Flexibility in the hips and knees can help prevent limitations in walking and bending, allowing you to easily navigate your environment. Imagine the liberation of getting up from a chair without hesitation or fear of discomfort.

Flexibility in these joints contributes significantly to balance, reducing the risk of falls and enhancing confidence in movement. It supports a life of independence and activity.

Maintaining shoulder and elbow range of motion is crucial for seniors as it directly impacts their ability to perform daily activities independently. The shoulders and elbows are integral for numerous basic tasks such as dressing, eating, grooming, and reaching for items, which become increasingly important as one ages. Limited mobility in these joints can lead to a reduced quality of life, as it might necessitate assistance for simple tasks, potentially causing a loss of autonomy and self-esteem.

Regular exercises that focus on preserving or enhancing shoulder and elbow flexibility can help mitigate stiffness, reduce arthritis pain, and prevent muscle atrophy that supports these joints. Additionally, having a good range of motion can help prevent falls by allowing for better balance and reaction when reaching or stabilizing oneself.

Flexibility is crucial for maintaining independence, enabling you to perform everyday tasks with ease. With increased flexibility, reaching overhead becomes effortless, reducing strain on the shoulders and back. Bending to pick up items from the floor is less taxing, which enhances safety and reduces the risk of falls. A flexible body moves gracefully through daily activities, supporting an active and independent lifestyle.

To safely progress your flexibility over time, focus on incrementally increasing the length and intensity of each stretch. Listen to your body's signals and avoid overexertion or discomfort. By practicing patience and consistency, you can gradually enhance your flexibility, supporting a life of mobility and independence.

Stretching routines should be tailored to individual capabilities, focusing on gentle, sustained stretches rather than aggressive or ballistic movements. Regular stretching is vital, as sporadic sessions will not yield long-term benefits. Incorporating stretching into daily routines can be an effective way to improve overall well-being

Interactive Element: Stretching Exercises

Utilize the following checklist to guide your stretching routine, ensuring you address all significant joints for comprehensive flexibility.

Performing these movements mindfully and carefully is crucial to preventing strain or injury. Avoid pushing through pain, as this can cause microtears in muscle tissue, tendinitis, or ligament strain. Gentle execution allows your body to adapt gradually. Each stretch targets areas prone to stiffness, providing a balanced approach to muscle and joint health.

SHOULDER STRETCH: Purpose- Relieves shoulder and upper back tension, improving posture and reducing shoulder pain.

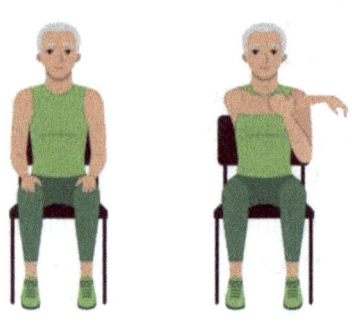

- Sit on a chair with your back supported.
- Reach one arm across your chest towards the opposite shoulder and use your other hand to gently press the elbow of the stretching arm closer to your chest.
- Hold for 20-30 seconds, then switch arms and repeat.
- Perform 3-5 sets.

SEATED HAMSTRING STRETCH: Purpose- Increases flexibility in the hamstrings, which can help with lower back pain and improve lower extremity mobility.

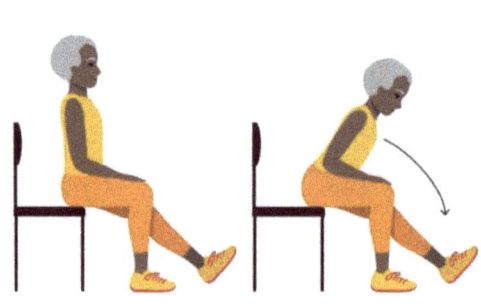

- Sit in the middle or towards the edge of the chair with one leg straight out in front of you and your toes pointing up.
- Lean forward slightly from your hips, keeping your back straight until you feel a stretch in the back of your thigh.
- Hold for 20-30 seconds.
- Switch legs and repeat.
- Perform 3-5 sets.

SEATED QUADRICEPS STRETCH: <u>Purpose</u>- Stretches the front thigh muscles, aiding knee and hip range of motion.

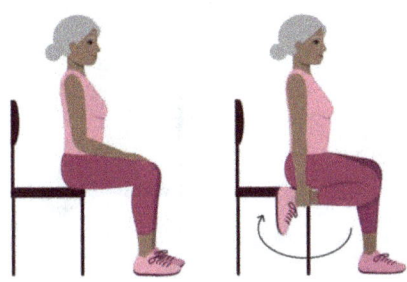

- Sit on the edge of your seat and slightly to one side, such as to the right.
- Bend the right knee, bring your heel towards your buttocks, and grab your ankle with the hand on the same side, or wrap a towel around it.
- Pull your ankle back until you feel a stretch in the front of your thigh.
- Hold for 20-30 seconds, then switch legs.
- Perform 3-5 sets.

SEATED GLUTEAL STRETCHES: <u>Purpose</u>- Relieves lower back pain, sciatica symptoms, and hip tension, improving overall hip mobility.

Stretch #1

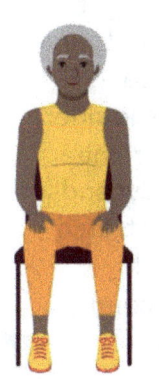
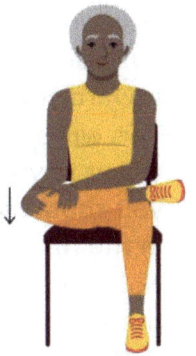

- Sit on a chair with your back supported.
- Cross your right leg over the left leg so your ankle rests on the left knee.
- Gently press down on the knee of the right leg, or lean forward slightly. You should feel a stretch in your right buttock and outer hip.
- Hold for 20-30 seconds, then switch to the other side.
- Perform 3-5 sets.

Modification: If you cannot cross one leg over the other due to significant inflexibility, do this instead:

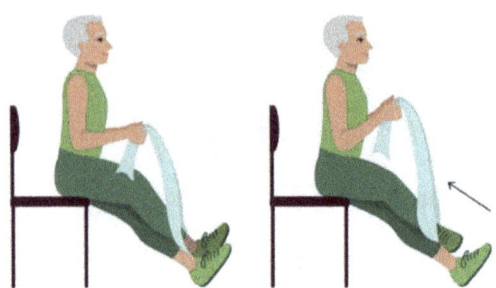

- Slightly extend the left leg.
- Place a towel around the ankle of the right leg.
- Cross the right ankle over the extended left ankle.
- Using the towel, gently slide your right ankle up the shin of the left leg as far as you can.
- Hold for 20-30 seconds, then switch sides.
- Perform 3-5 sets.

Gluteal Stretch #2:

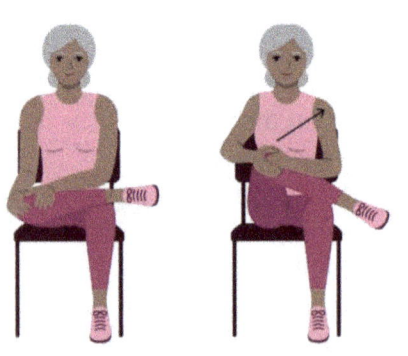

- Sit on a chair with your back supported.
- Cross your right leg over the left knee so your right calf muscle rests on the left knee.
- Gently grasp your right knee with both hands and pull your right knee toward your left shoulder.
- This will bring your knee closer to your body, and you should feel a stretch in the right buttock.
- Hold for 20-30 seconds, then switch sides.
- Perform 3-5 sets.

Modification: If you cannot cross one leg over to place the calf on the opposite knee due to significant inflexibility, do this instead:

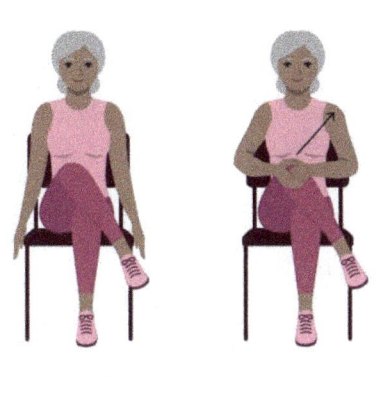

- ○ Cross the right leg fully over the left leg as much as you can.
- ○ This may cause stretching in your gluteal area; if so, hold this position for 20-30 seconds.
- ○ If you can, pull your right knee toward your left shoulder. This will bring your knee closer to your body, and you should feel a stretch in the right buttock.
- ○ Hold for 20-30 seconds, then switch sides.
- ○ Perform 3-5 sets.

SEATED CALF STRETCH: <u>Purpose</u>- Prevents or alleviates calf tightness affecting ankle range of motion, walking, and balance.

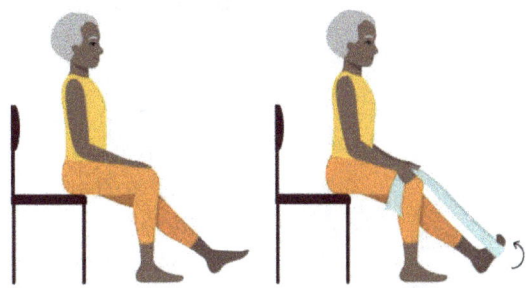

- ○ Sit toward the edge of your seat with one leg extended in front of you.
- ○ Flex your foot so your toes come towards you, keeping your heel on the ground. Enhance the stretch by placing a towel around the ball of your foot, holding the ends of the towel, and pulling your foot toward you to stretch the calf.
- ○ Hold for 20-30 seconds, then switch legs.
- ○ Perform 3-5 sets.

SEATED LOW BACK STRETCH: <u>Purpose-</u> targets the lower back, helping to alleviate tension, improve flexibility.

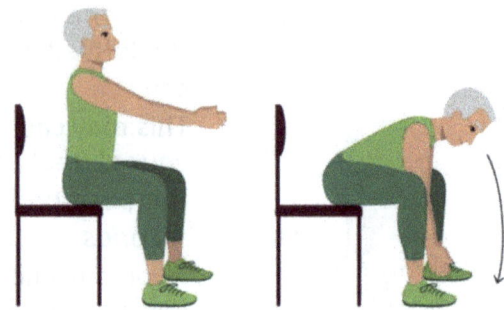

- Sit toward the edge of a chair with your feet apart.
- Bring your hands together and slowly bend forward toward the ground between your legs, down as comfortably as possible without forcing the stretch. Bend from your hips, not your waist.
- Hold for 20-30 seconds and return to the starting position.
- Perform 3-5 sets.

SEATED TORSO SIDE STRETCH: <u>Purpose-</u> Increases spine flexibility, reduces back pain.

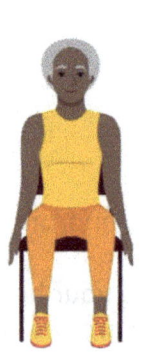 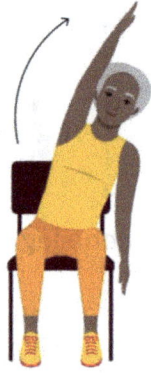

- Sit on a chair with or without your back supported
- Slowly lean to one side, extending the opposite arm over your head if comfortable, feeling a stretch along the side of your torso.
- Hold for 20-30 seconds.
- Return to the center and repeat on the other side.
- Perform 3-5 sets.

SEATED NECK STRETCHES: <u>Purpose</u>: Alleviates neck stiffness and tension, promoting better head movement.

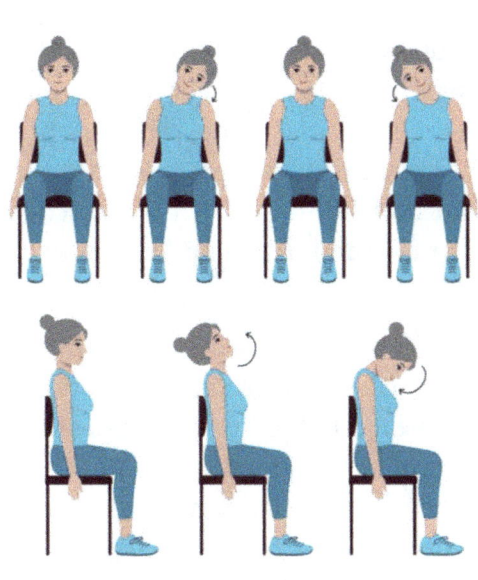

- Sit on a chair with your back supported
- Tilt your head to one side, bringing your ear towards your shoulder until you feel a stretch. Hold for 20-30 seconds.
- Return to the center and tilt to the other side.
- Next, gently tuck your chin to your chest. Hold for 20-30 seconds.
- Then look up towards the ceiling. Hold for 20-30 seconds.
- Perform 3-5 sets each.

Progression: You can provide additional stretch to the neck muscles by pulling gently on your head during each tilt if shoulder range of motion permits.

The holistic benefits of incorporating these gentle movements into your routine extend beyond physical relief. Regular practice can improve one's mood, and reduced pain levels translate into greater ease in performing daily tasks. The psychological impact of this newfound freedom can be profound, fostering a sense of empowerment and independence. As you experience less pain, your confidence in your abilities may increase, encouraging you to explore new activities and engage more fully in life. This overall enhancement of well-being underscores the value of gentle exercise in managing pain and stiffness.

9.3 Reduce Stiffness Throughout the Day

Developing a structured stretching routine is a practical way to combat stiffness and maintain joint health. Start your day with morning stretches that gradually awaken your body. While still in bed, you might begin with gentle supine stretches that transition into sitting poses, easing your body into the day's activities. This gentle approach alleviates morning stiffness and sets a positive tone for the hours ahead. As evening approaches, incorporate wind-down stretches that promote relaxation and prepare your body for restful sleep. Stretching exercises help release the day's accumulated tension and encourage a calm, peaceful state of mind.

Incorporating stretching during the day can prevent stiffness buildup and keep your muscles limber. Gentle head tilts, for instance, relieve neck tension, a common issue exacerbated by prolonged sitting or poor posture. Shoulder shrugs offer another effective way to release tension in the upper body. Wrist and ankle circles can alleviate joint stiffness and improve range of motion.

Gardening and household chores offer a prime opportunity to incorporate stretching into daily activities. Before you begin, perform gentle stretches that prepare your body for the physical demands of gardening or cleaning. Stretching your back, shoulders, and legs can prevent strain and enhance your enjoyment of the activity. Remember to pause occasionally for a quick stretch before you engage in these tasks.

Stretching during daily activities, such as while watching television commercials or waiting for the kettle to boil, provides ideal opportunities to engage in brief exercises that promote flexibility and joint health. Before exercising or engaging in physical activities, use stretching as a warm-up to prepare your muscles and joints. Afterward, stretch to cool down, helping your body recover and relax.

Chapter 10: Creating a Sustainable Exercise Habit

Reflecting on my experiences with clients, it's clear that many seniors struggle to maintain a consistent exercise regimen. Retired professionals often approach physical activity with the same methodical mindset they applied to their careers; yet, they face significant barriers, including limited time, pain, and diminished energy. I often hear from patients who were once very active, such as former football players or dancers, reminiscing about their past. These stories highlight a stark contrast between their youthful vigor and current physical limitations, illustrating the challenge of adapting exercise habits to fit new life stages. By understanding this transition, we can better address how to overcome these barriers, ensuring that exercise remains a fulfilling and sustainable part of their lives.

A senior living alone might find it particularly challenging to maintain self-motivation for an exercise program due to several factors. It's easy to lose enthusiasm or skip sessions when exercising without the companionship or accountability that comes with working out with others. The quiet solitude can amplify feelings of isolation, making the effort to start exercising feel daunting. Moreover, physical limitations or health concerns might make previously enjoyable activities less feasible, leading to discouragement. The absence of immediate support to celebrate small victories or push through tough days can diminish the drive to continue. Daily routines might not naturally include time for physical activity, and the motivation to stick to a regular exercise schedule can wane without external cues or social interactions.

Weather-related challenges can significantly impact a senior's ability to maintain a consistent exercise routine, especially when outdoor activities are preferred. In regions with harsh winters or scorching summers, the elements can pose significant threats to health and safety. Extreme cold can lead to risks such as slippery conditions, which increase the likelihood of falls. In contrast, extreme heat can cause dehydration or exacerbate cardiovascular issues. These conditions discourage outdoor exercise, and if no alternatives exist, can lead to a sedentary lifestyle.

This chapter examines the common challenges seniors face when trying to maintain an exercise program. It discusses how to transform challenges into opportunities for adaptation and provides practical strategies to help seniors maintain a regular and satisfying exercise routine, regardless of external conditions or personal energy levels.

10.1 Overcoming Common Exercise Barriers

Identifying the barriers to physical activity is the first step in establishing a lasting exercise practice. Many seniors struggle with a perceived lack of time, often overwhelmed by the demands of daily life. Balancing family responsibilities, social engagements, and personal care can leave little room for exercise. Low energy levels, a common issue that arises with age, can be challenging, and fatigue can diminish motivation, making it difficult to engage in physical activities.

Overcoming perceived barriers to exercise starts with reframing time management and energy conservation. One strategy to overcome the time barrier is to integrate physical activity into daily routines in small, manageable chunks, rather than dedicating long sessions. For instance, you can break up exercise into short, frequent sessions, such as a 10- or 15-minute seated strengthening exercise session after meals or light stretching during commercial breaks. Integrating exercise into daily routines allows you to seamlessly incorporate physical activity into your day by identifying pockets of time that align with existing activities. This approach not only maximizes time efficiency but also reinforces the habit of regular exercise.

Creating indoor alternatives, such as chair yoga, using a stationary bike, or walking in the mall, helps ensure that exercise remains a consistent part of your life, even in unfavorable weather conditions.

Addressing low energy involves understanding one's body rhythms and exercising when energy levels are naturally higher, like late morning or early afternoon. You can conserve energy by performing chair exercises or by utilizing an assistive device while exercising, which provides physical benefits without overwhelming the body. Additionally, setting realistic goals that account for daily life demands can reduce the pressure to perform, making exercise seem less like a chore and more like a part of daily life.

For individuals living alone who may struggle with self-motivation, utilizing technology such as fitness apps or smart devices that remind, track, and celebrate achievements can be incredibly supportive. Joining a fitness class or group specifically designed for seniors can significantly boost exercise motivation by providing a supportive community where members encourage one another. This social interaction makes workouts more enjoyable and creates a sense of accountability, helping seniors consistently stick to their fitness routines.

Educating oneself about the tangible benefits of exercise for health and longevity can reinforce commitment and transform exercise from a daunting task into an achievable and rewarding endeavor. Additionally, varying the exercise routine to keep it interesting and focusing on exercises that have immediate feel-good effects, like improved balance or reduced pain, helps sustain interest.

Building mental resilience is crucial in maintaining an exercise routine amidst life's challenges. Celebrating small achievements can significantly boost motivation, no matter how minor they may seem. Recognizing progress in balance, strength, or flexibility reinforces the benefits of regular exercise, encouraging continued effort. Setting realistic expectations is equally important, as it prevents discouragement. Recognize that progress may be gradual, and setbacks are a natural part of the process. You cultivate resilience and perseverance by maintaining a positive outlook and focusing on incremental improvements.

Professional guidance can provide valuable support and motivation, especially when facing barriers to exercise. Consulting with fitness or healthcare professionals offers personalized advice tailored to your unique needs and goals. Engaging a personal trainer can introduce new techniques and routines, enhancing the effectiveness and enjoyment of your exercise program. Personal trainers provide accountability, ensuring you stay committed to your routine. Attending fitness workshops or classes introduces a social element, fostering a sense of community and support. These interactions enrich your exercise experience and provide opportunities to learn and grow alongside others with similar goals.

Reflection Section: Identifying Your Exercise Barriers

Take a moment to reflect on the barriers that prevent you from maintaining a consistent exercise routine. Consider the following questions:

- What specific obstacles prevent you from engaging in regular physical activity?
- How do these barriers impact your motivation and energy levels?
- What strategies can you implement to overcome these challenges?
- How can you integrate exercise into your daily routine amidst these obstacles?

By identifying your unique barriers and devising a plan to address them, you empower yourself to create a sustainable exercise habit. Through resilience, adaptability, and support, you can transform challenges into opportunities. Incorporating these strategies fosters a resilient mindset, enabling you to navigate obstacles with confidence and determination. Addressing barriers head-on and embracing adaptability lays the foundation for a sustainable exercise habit.

10.2 Setting Achievable Fitness Goals

Setting achievable fitness goals for seniors embarking on an exercise journey is like planting stepping stones across a river. Each stone represents a clear, reachable goal that guides you safely to the other side, where better health and vitality await. These goals transform vague ideas into clear, manageable steps, making the route to better health much easier to follow.

Setting realistic targets lays a foundation that keeps motivation and success within reach.

Breaking Goals Down: Break down large goals into smaller, more manageable steps. This strategy makes the journey less overwhelming and celebrates each small victory, keeping you motivated.

Personalizing Your Goals: Consider your physical state, limitations, and what you want to achieve. Do you want better flexibility, improved balance, fewer falls, or more stamina? Tailor your goals to match these needs. For instance, if balance is your focus, include specific balance exercises a few times a week. This personal approach crafts a unique roadmap for your fitness journey.

Short and Long-Term Goals: Set immediate goals, such as doing strength exercises four days a week for the next two weeks. These give you quick wins to aim for. Then, set broader, long-term goals, such as increasing your overall strength over a six-month period. Both provide direction and a sense of urgency, pushing you to keep moving forward.

Making Goals Engaging: Imagine the joy of achieving these goals. Picture yourself moving quickly and enjoying your daily life more because of your improved health. No matter how small, each step is a step towards that vibrant life.

By approaching fitness this way, you're not just exercising; you're embarking on a journey tailored just for you, celebrating each step toward a healthier, more active lifestyle.

The SMART Criteria for Effective Goal-Setting in Fitness

The SMART criteria—Specific, Measurable, Achievable, Relevant, and Time-bound—provide a powerful framework for setting fitness goals. Here's how each component works:

Specific: Your goals need to be clear and precise. Instead of a vague goal like "exercise more," you might say, "I will do core strengthening exercises every other day." Specificity removes ambiguity and defines your goals.

Measurable: You need to track your progress. For instance, set a goal like "increase the number of repetitions in each exercise session every two weeks." This provides you with concrete benchmarks to track your progress and celebrate your achievements.

Achievable: Goals should be realistic, considering your current fitness level and lifestyle. Setting an attainable goal encourages success rather than frustration.

Relevant: Ensure your goals align with your priorities and values. Ask yourself, "Why is this goal important to me?"

Time-bound: Add deadlines to your goals, such as "I will master three new poses within the next month." This creates urgency and focus.

By making your fitness goals SMART, you'll create a path to rewarding and fulfilling success. This will transform exercise into something more than a routine—it becomes a journey of self-discovery and improvement.

The benefits of goal-setting go beyond physical health. Clear goals fuel commitment and perseverance, giving you a sense of purpose and direction. Visualizing the benefits of reaching these goals creates a mental picture of success that keeps you motivated, even when obstacles appear. Celebrating even the smallest victories uplifts your spirit and strengthens your dedication.

Every little achievement, no matter how minor, reminds you of your progress and potential, fueling your drive to keep going. Goal-setting isn't merely about getting to a finish line; it's about the journey of growth and self-improvement. By setting achievable fitness goals, you are taking charge of your health and well-being.

Reflect on this: What does success look like in your fitness journey? What small victory could you celebrate today?

10.3 Keeping Motivation High with Diverse Routines

Maintaining motivation in your exercise routine requires more than willpower; it's about variety and engagement. Think of your fitness plan as a recipe that benefits from diverse ingredients. You can turn your routine into an exciting adventure by incorporating activities such as swimming, walking, biking, and gentle strength training. Engaging different muscle groups and challenging your body in new ways prevents boredom and boosts motivation. The freshness this brings keeps your mind and body invigorated, sparking enthusiasm and commitment.

The psychological benefits of a varied exercise routine are significant. Changing activities weekly, from chair strengthening to standing exercises or introducing chair cardio or stationary biking, keeps the routine fresh. This approach reduces monotony, increases anticipation, and stimulates mental engagement as you challenge your coordination and balance. This mental workout is just as crucial as physical exercise and enhances cognitive function.

Assigning specific activities to certain days can provide predictability, making it easier to form new habits. Joining group classes adds another layer of variety, offering social interaction that can be motivating. The collective energy and learning new exercises in such settings can broaden your fitness repertoire and keep you inspired.

Engaging in activities you enjoy and tailoring your routine to reflect your interests and goals is essential. This personalization makes exercise more enjoyable and rewarding, reinforcing your commitment. Keep an open mind for exploration and experimentation, letting your interests guide your choices. This approach creates a sense of excitement and anticipation, fueling your motivation to remain active.

Moreover, a varied routine enables you to tailor exercises to your physical needs. If you're aiming for flexibility, yoga and stretching are essential. For those focusing on improving balance, standing chair balance exercises can be incredibly beneficial. Strength training with weights or resistance bands helps maintain muscle mass. By aligning your exercises with your personal goals, each session becomes a step toward achieving your health objectives, boosting your motivation, and enhancing your overall satisfaction.

10.4 Overcoming Exercise Plateaus

Encountering an exercise plateau can feel like slamming into an invisible barrier, halting progress. However, understanding what an exercise plateau is can be transformative if you're committed to your routine. A plateau occurs when your body has adapted to your current workout level, leading to a standstill in progress despite your consistent efforts. This stagnation is a shared experience, often because our routines become too familiar or lack the necessary intensity to further challenge us.

Recognizing you're at a plateau involves noticing that the improvements in strength, endurance, or flexibility you once enjoyed have now leveled off. Setting realistic expectations about the time it might take to see changes is crucial. Fitness progress isn't a straight path; sometimes, it meanders, and patience is your greatest ally. Generally, you might see noticeable improvements after several weeks as your body adjusts to the new physical demands. However, if your exercise habits are inconsistent, this can worsen plateaus, as your body cannot fully adapt to a changing regimen.

When you feel stuck, it's time to ask yourself: What can I do differently? Breaking through a plateau often requires some creativity or a change in approach:

Increase Intensity: It may be time to lift heavier weights, move faster, or add more resistance. Small increments can make a big difference.

Change Your Routine: Introduce new exercises or alter the sequence of your current ones. Cross-training, such as chair yoga for strength and balance or swimming for low-impact cardio, can rejuvenate your routine.

Rest and Recovery: Sometimes, a plateau indicates that your body requires additional recovery time. Incorporating active recovery days or ensuring enough sleep can reset your progress.

Nutrition and Hydration: Often overlooked, your diet plays a crucial role in achieving your fitness goals. Ensure you're fueling your body correctly for recovery and performance.

Mental Reset: To tackle the psychological aspect of plateaus, engage in mental exercises like visualization or meditation. Believing in your ability to overcome this hurdle is as crucial as the physical effort.

Seek Inspiration: Join a class, find a workout buddy, or discover fitness videos to inspire you. Sometimes, the motivation to push through comes from external sources.

Remember, what worked for someone else might not work for you, so be open to experimenting with different strategies. Reflect on past successes or failures with plateaus; what lessons can you draw from them? How have you adapted before, and what new techniques might you try this time?

By actively addressing these questions and adapting your approach, you can break through that plateau and reignite your journey toward better health, strength, and vitality. It's not just about pushing harder; it's about being more thoughtful, ensuring that each step of your fitness journey is as rewarding as it's challenging.

Chapter 11: Promoting Relaxation and Stress Relief

As a physical therapist, I've encountered many patients dealing with pain or stress during therapy. For those struggling with the physical and emotional toll of their conditions, simple tasks can feel overwhelming. One common strategy I introduce is deep breathing as a relaxation tool. It has proven to be a revelation for numerous patients. Through structured breathing exercises, they find ways to manage their pain and emotions, reducing anxiety and promoting a sense of peace. These experiences demonstrate the transformative power of controlled breathing, which can significantly alleviate pain, ease anxiety, and promote relaxation. This chapter explores how to integrate these techniques into your daily life, thereby enhancing both your mental and physical well-being.

11.1 Relaxation Techniques

Breathing is an innate function, yet it becomes a powerful ally against stress when harnessed with intention. Among the foundational techniques is abdominal breathing, also known as diaphragmatic breathing, as discussed in Chapter 1.5. This technique involves sitting comfortably, placing one hand on your chest and the other on your abdomen. As you inhale slowly through your nose, let your abdomen expand, feeling the hand on your stomach rise more than the one on your chest. This deep, deliberate breath fills your lungs more completely, promoting a sense of relaxation. Take your time with the exhale, making it longer than the inhale, as your abdomen contracts, and you push the air out entirely through pursed lips. This method calms the mind and engages the diaphragm, encouraging full oxygen exchange and reducing tension.

For best results, practice this technique for a few minutes daily, gradually increasing the duration as you become more comfortable. Incorporating it into your routine can enhance its benefits, helping you manage stress more effectively. Try it now, and notice how your body responds to this simple yet powerful practice.

Another effective technique is deep breathing with slow counts. This exercise begins by sitting or lying in a relaxed position. Inhale deeply through your nose, counting slowly to four, and allow your lungs to fill. Hold your breath for a count of four, then exhale through your mouth, releasing all tension with the breath. This rhythmic pattern slows the breathing rate, promoting a state of calm. By focusing on the count, your mind shifts away from stressors, anchoring you in the present moment. Try this technique right now to experience its calming effects.

Physiologically, these breathing exercises activate the parasympathetic nervous system, which governs the body's rest and digestion functions. When engaged, this system counters the fight-or-flight response triggered by stress, reducing heart rate and blood pressure. This state of relaxation enables the body to repair and restore itself, fostering a sense of well-being. Moreover, increased oxygenation of the bloodstream and brain enhances cognitive clarity and focus. As the brain receives more oxygen, it functions more efficiently, supporting mental tasks and emotional regulation. This physiological shift underscores the profound impact of controlled breathing on stress reduction. The next time you feel stressed, try these breathing exercises to activate your body's natural relaxation response and experience the difference.

Incorporating breathing techniques into everyday activities helps it become a natural stress response, enhancing resilience and adaptability. Deep breathing can immediately relieve acute stress, helping you regain control and composure. Additionally, using these exercises to manage shortness of breath during physical activity ensures that your body receives adequate oxygen, supporting endurance and stamina. Over time, improved lung capacity contributes to overall physical health, enabling more confident and efficient engagement in physical activity.

Regular deep breathing exercises enhance emotional regulation, enabling you to manage stressors and respond to challenges with poise. This emotional stability translates to improved relationships and social interactions as you navigate life's demands with a balanced mindset. Furthermore, the mental clarity and focus gained from these exercises bolster cognitive performance, supporting tasks that require concentration and attention.

11.2 Add Relaxation into Daily Routines

As we navigate the demands of daily life, setting aside dedicated time for relaxation is a vital practice. Consider identifying specific times each day to unwind, whether in the morning to start calmly or in the evening to release the day's tension. This dedicated time can be brief, such as ten minutes, or extended to an hour, depending on your schedule and needs. Over time, these moments of calm permeate your entire day, allowing you to approach tasks with a clearer, more focused mind.

Combining relaxation with existing activities can seamlessly integrate tranquility into one's life. For instance, while performing household chores, listen to calming music to make the task more enjoyable and turn it into a calming ritual. The gentle melodies soothe the mind, reduce stress, and create a peaceful atmosphere.

One of the most notable benefits of relation is a reduction in chronic stress levels, which can otherwise contribute to health issues like heart disease, hypertension, and a weakened immune system. By incorporating relaxation into your daily routine, you can mitigate these risks, ultimately fostering a healthier and more resilient body. Improved sleep quality and duration often follow as your mind unwinds, making it easier to fall asleep and deepen your rest. This restorative sleep enhances cognitive function, mood, and energy levels, preparing you to tackle each day with renewed vigor.

Integrating gentle movement, such as stretching, into your routine offers a powerful means of alleviating stress and promoting relaxation. Light physical activities help release tension that accumulates in the body throughout the day, easing physical discomfort and uplifting the spirit, thereby fostering an improved mood and increased energy levels. Each movement invites calm, counteracting daily stress. Gentle exercises bridge the physical and mental, allowing you to address stress holistically.

Treat these moments as non-negotiable appointments with yourself, prioritizing your well-being. Additionally, relaxation and mindfulness apps can provide structure and guidance. Many offer reminders and exercises, making it easier to maintain your routine.

They serve as convenient resources, guiding you through practices that promote calmness and mindfulness and support your mental and physical well-being.

11.3 Mindfulness Practices for Seniors

Rooted in ancient traditions, mindfulness has become a valuable tool for reducing stress and promoting well-being. At its core, mindfulness involves embracing the present moment without judgment. This focus allows you to step back from the constant chatter of the mind and engage more deeply with your surroundings and inner self. In today's fast-paced world, where distractions abound, mindfulness is an anchor, bringing clarity and calm. Concentrating on the present can reduce stress and anxiety, fostering a sense of peace and balance. Mindfulness isn't just about awareness; it's about acceptance and fully experiencing each moment. This practice can shift your perspective, leading to better stress management, improved health, and reduced pain.

For those new to mindfulness, starting with simple exercises can be both practical and rewarding. Mindful eating is an excellent introduction to this practice. By paying attention to the flavors, textures, and aromas of your food, you can enhance your enjoyment and develop a greater appreciation for meals. This exercise encourages you to eat more slowly, savoring each bite and promoting better digestion. It also helps you recognize hunger and fullness cues, supporting healthier eating habits. The next time you sit down for a meal, try practicing mindful eating and see how it alters your experience.

Another effective technique is the body scan meditation. This form of mindful meditation involves lying down or sitting comfortably and focusing on each part of the body. As you mentally travel from your toes to your head, notice areas of tension or relaxation. This exercise heightens awareness of bodily sensations, allowing you to release tension and experience relaxation. By fostering a deeper connection with your body, the body scan promotes a sense of comfort and peace.

Mindfulness can significantly alter one's mental state and how one experiences pain and discomfort. Focusing on positive or neutral sensations within one's body can shift one's focus, often decreasing pain intensity and lessening its impact. Mindfulness doesn't aim to eliminate pain or stress but changes how you relate to these experiences, making them more manageable. Over time, this practice can improve mental and physical health outcomes by reducing stress. It teaches you to live more fully in each moment, fostering a deeper connection with yourself and promoting a balanced, serene approach to life's ups and downs.

Including mindfulness in daily life is straightforward and doesn't require a significant amount of time or effort. Short, frequent sessions can be as beneficial as longer ones. Integrate mindfulness into routine activities, such as brushing your teeth or walking, by focusing entirely on the task. Through this process, you learn to appreciate each moment, navigate life's complexities more effectively, and discover a path to increased awareness and serenity, thereby enriching both body and mind.

As we conclude our exploration of relaxation and stress relief practices, it is evident that incorporating these techniques into your daily routine offers profound benefits. Reducing stress, improving sleep, and enhancing overall well-being build a foundation for a balanced and fulfilling life.

Chapter 12: Inspiring Others: Sharing Your Journey

Every senior has a unique journey with exercise and chair yoga, filled with personal victories and insights that can inspire and empower others. Reflecting on your path helps you recognize how far you've come and highlights the obstacles you've overcome. When you share these stories, you contribute to a rich tapestry of community wisdom and support.

Sharing your story in community newsletters is a great way to connect with those who may be unsure or unaware of the benefits of chair yoga. Your narrative can act as a guiding light, leading others towards health and independence.

Platforms like social media and online forums are perfect for spreading your insights. By sharing your journey online, you can ignite motivation and inspire a broader audience to adopt a healthier lifestyle, taking their first steps toward a healthier life. Your story could be the spark that lights up someone else's path to wellness.

The strength of community and mutual support is invaluable. Sharing your experiences affirms your place within a collective movement towards better health and well-being. This shared space fosters connections and nurtures motivation. When you share your journey, you inspire others to try chair yoga, encouraging them to join classes or groups. This collective involvement enriches the experience, creating a sense of camaraderie and shared goals. The community then becomes a pillar of support, providing encouragement and accountability. Engaging with others on this journey helps create an environment where everyone feels supported, inspired, and motivated to reach their full potential. Here's your call to action:

Share Your Story: Write about your experience with chair yoga in your community's newsletter or share it on social media.

Join the Conversation: Engage with others in online forums or local groups to exchange stories and tips.

Be a Beacon: Let your journey light the way for someone else, showing them how transformative chair yoga and other forms of exercise can be.

Creating platforms where seniors can share and learn from each other fosters collective inspiration. Whether through local or virtual meet-ups, these gatherings provide a space for supportive storytelling, either casually through discussion or more formally with guest speakers or workshops. Collaborating with community centers can expand these opportunities, providing additional resources and access to chair yoga. These environments foster a culture of shared growth and empowerment, where inspiration and support are abundant.

Leverage various tools to enhance your storytelling. A reflection section in your journal can clarify thoughts and emotions as you prepare to share. A checklist of key themes ensures your narrative stays focused and impactful. Enhance your story with visual elements, such as photographs or simple infographics, to vividly illustrate your achievements. These tools enrich communication for the storyteller and the audience, fostering a dynamic exchange of ideas and inspiration.

Remember, your story is uniquely valuable. Your journey, with its insights and achievements, adds to the narrative of resilience in the senior community and positions you as a participant and a leader in this transformative movement. Your story matters. Tell it, share it, and watch the ripple effect of inspiration spread.

Now that you've got all the tools to boost your balance, strength, and flexibility, it's time to spread the word and help others discover the same benefits.

By sharing your honest thoughts about this book, you can help other seniors find the resources to start their journey with chair exercises.

Thank you for your help. We keep the senior exercise community alive by passing on our knowledge, and you're helping me do just that.

S. Carroll, MPT

Conclusion

As you reach the end of this book, let's reflect on the transformative journey that chair yoga offers. We've explored the multifaceted benefits of chair yoga, specifically tailored for seniors, which enhance physical strength, balance, and flexibility, key to maintaining independence and improving quality of life. You can experience reduced pain, increased mobility, and enhanced well-being by incorporating simple, structured exercises into your daily routine. This practice also fosters a sense of control over your physical health, empowering you to navigate daily tasks with renewed confidence and ease.

This book offers practical guidance on creating a safe exercise environment at home, utilizing household items as tools, and understanding the importance of nutrition and hydration in complementing your practice. Each chapter guides you through the steps for practical and enjoyable exercise sessions, from foundational breathing techniques that promote relaxation to advanced positions and adaptations for those with limited mobility. We've also explored how to listen to your body, ensuring each movement feels supportive and sustainable, allowing you to progress at a pace that suits you.

As a home health physical therapist with over a decade of experience, I've witnessed exercise transform lives, often turning moments of frustration into opportunities for growth. I encourage you to take your first step toward integrating chair yoga into your routine. Start with exercises that resonate with you, address specific areas of discomfort or limitation, and gradually expand your practice to explore new movements. Consistency is key; set realistic goals that align with your lifestyle and track your progress with journaling or checklists. Even small, regular efforts can yield significant benefits over time, improving your physical capabilities and overall sense of vitality.

You're not alone on this journey. Countless seniors have shared their success stories, overcoming challenges such as chronic pain, stiffness, or a fear of falling, and achieving remarkable transformations that ripple into other areas of their lives. Remember, every small step in your chair yoga journey is a victory worth celebrating, whether holding a pose a little longer, feeling less pain in your joints, or simply enjoying a moment of calm during your practice.

I am grateful for the opportunity to guide you through this process. Your dedication to enhancing your health is commendable, and I am honored to support you as you explore the possibilities of chair yoga. Embrace the changes it brings to your life, knowing you have the tools to succeed, from the exercises to the strategies for staying motivated and engaged.

As you move forward, carry the encouragement and support from this book. May your journey with chair yoga be fulfilling and transformative, opening doors to new experiences and connections. Approach each session with an open heart and a willingness to explore new possibilities, experimenting with different times of day or settings to find what feels most enriching. Your commitment to this practice is a testament to your strength and resilience, and it has the potential to inspire others in your community. Thank you for entrusting me with your journey toward a healthier, more vibrant life.

References

Effect of Chair Yoga Therapy on Functional Fitness and ...
https://pmc.ncbi.nlm.nih.gov/articles/PMC10094373/

How to Create a Senior-Friendly Exercise Space at Home
https://www.seniorhelpers.com/va/stafford/resources/blogs/how-to-create-a-senior-friendly-exercise-space-at-home/

12 Everyday Household Items That Double as Gym ...
https://www.cnet.com/health/fitness/12-everyday-household-items-for-your-workouts/

Breathing Exercises https://www.lung.org/lung-health-diseases/wellness/breathing-exercises

Yoga: A flexible way to enhance heart health
https://www.health.harvard.edu/heart-health/yoga-a-flexible-way-to-enhance-heart-health

Yoga for Arthritis: Benefits, Poses, and Tips to Get Started
https://www.goodrx.com/well-being/movement-exercise/yoga-for-arthritis

Exercising with osteoporosis: Stay active the safe way
https://www.mayoclinic.org/diseases-conditions/osteoporosis/in-depth/osteoporosis/art-20044989

Physical Activity Benefits for Adults 65 or Older
https://www.cdc.gov/physical-activity-basics/health-benefits/older-adults.html

Protein Consumption and the Elderly: What Is the Optimal ...
https://pmc.ncbi.nlm.nih.gov/articles/PMC4924200/

How to Stay Hydrated: A Guide for Older Adults
https://www.ncoa.org/article/how-to-stay-hydrated-for-better-health/

National Institutes of Health. (n.d.). Vitamin D. Office of Dietary Supplements. ods.od.nih.gov/factsheets/VitaminD-HealthProfessional/

Pre- and Post-Workout Nutrition: What to Eat and When ...
https://www.lifetimedaily.com/pre-and-post-workout-nutrition-for-older-adults/

How to Detect and Prevent Malnutrition in Seniors
https://www.ncoa.org/article/10-ways-malnutrition-can-impact-your-health-and-6-steps-to-prevent-it/

Chair yoga for seniors: Benefits and poses for beginners
https://www.medicalnewstoday.com/articles/chair-yoga-for-seniors

The Best Exercise Equipment for Seniors, Tested
https://www.verywellfit.com/best-exercise-equipment-for-seniors-7563564.

Protein Intake and Muscle Function in Older Adults - PMC
https://pmc.ncbi.nlm.nih.gov/articles/PMC4394186/

How to Stay Hydrated: A Guide for Older Adults
https://www.ncoa.org/article/how-to-stay-hydrated-for-better-health/

Exercise and Physical Activity Worksheets
https://www.nia.nih.gov/health/exercise-and-physical-activity/exercise-and-physical-activity-worksheets

Goal Setting for Seniors: Why It Is Important, Tips, & ...
https://www.pacificangelshomecare.com/blog/goal-setting-for-seniors/

The Reasons Why Seniors Need Fitness Trackers For Their ...
https://www.terrabellaseniorliving.com/senior-living-blog/the-reasons-why-seniors-need-fitness-trackers-for-their-exercise-programs.

The Best Health Monitoring Fitness Trackers for ...
https://villagegreenseniorliving.com/news/the-best-health-monitoring-fitness-trackers-for-seniors-2024/

Stretching for Seniors (and Why It's Important)
https://www.orlincohen.com/news/stretching-for-seniors-and-why-its-important/

5 Joint Mobility Exercises to Improve Flexibility and Function
https://www.healthline.com/health/fitness-exercise/joint-mobility-exercises

Hyaluronan and synovial joint: function, distribution and healing
https://pubmed.ncbi.nlm.nih.gov/24678248/

Six tips for safe stretches https://www.health.harvard.edu/staying-healthy/six-tips-for-safe-stretches

Fall Prevention: Balance and Strength Exercises for Older ...
https://www.hopkinsmedicine.org/health/wellness-and-prevention/fall-prevention-exercises

Seated exercise may improve cognition in older adults ...
https://www.mcmasteroptimalaging.org/full-article/es/seated-exercise-improve-cognition-older-adults-health-condition-impairment-3045.

Mindfulness in Fall Prevention https://www.mindful.org/mindfulness-in-fall-prevention/

Chair Yoga: How To Teach Yoga For Restricted Mobility https://www.arhantayoga.org/blog/chair-yoga-how-to-teach-yoga-for-restricted-mobility/

The Effect of Chair-Based Exercise on Physical Function in ... https://pmc.ncbi.nlm.nih.gov/articles/PMC7920319/

5 Safe balance exercises for seniors who use a walker https://www.caregiversolutions.ca/health-and-wellness/5-safe-balance-exercises-for-seniors-who-use-a-walker/

Exercising with arthritis: Improve your joint pain and stiffness https://www.mayoclinic.org/diseases-conditions/arthritis/in-depth/arthritis/art-20047971

4 Breathing Exercises for Older Adults To Cope with Stress https://sunhealthcommunities.org/helpful-tools/articles/4-breathing-exercises-older-adults-cope-stress/

A qualitative study of older adults' perspectives on initiating exercise and mindfulness practice- *https://bmcgeriatr.biomedcentral.com/articles/10.1186/s12877-019-1375-9*

Exercising to Relax - Harvard Health Publishing https://www.health.harvard.edu/staying-healthy/exercising-to-relax

Incorporating Mindfulness and Meditation in Seniors' Daily ... https://celebrateseniorliving.org/2023/09/25/incorporating-mindfulness-and-meditation-in-seniors-daily-routine/

Overcoming Barriers to Physical Activity While Aging https://extension.sdstate.edu/overcoming-barriers-physical-activity-while-aging

S.M.A.R.T. goals for seniors! https://eventide.org/smart-goals-for-seniors/

The Importance of Exercise Variety for Seniors https://www.ahealthiermichigan.org/stories/health-and-wellness/the-importance-of-exercise-variety-for-seniors

10 Tips for Powering Through Plateaus https://www.acefitness.org/resources/everyone/blog/5851/10-tips-for-powering-through-plateaus

Effect of Chair Yoga Therapy on Functional Fitness and ...
https://pmc.ncbi.nlm.nih.gov/articles/PMC10094373/

Chair Yoga Saved Me From A Wheelchair
https://www.womansworld.com/wellness/chair-yoga-for-seniors

Impact of Yoga on cognition and mental health among elderly
https://pubmed.ncbi.nlm.nih.gov/32951703/

Adapting Exercises for Seniors with Limited Mobility
https://allamericanatwrentham.com/adapting-exercises-for-seniors-with-limited-mobility/

Arthritis Foundation. (n.d.). 8 ways exercise helps joints. Arthritis.org. https://www.arthritis.org/health-wellness/healthy-living/physical-activity/getting-started/8-ways-exercise-helps-joints

Argilés, J. M., Busquets, S., & López-Soriano, F. J. (2005). The pivotal role of cytokines in muscle wasting during cancer. International Journal of Biochemistry & Cell Biology, 37(8), 1609-1619.

Chernoff, R. (2004). Protein and older adults. Journal of the American College of Nutrition, 23(6 Suppl), 627S-630S.

Evans, W. J. (1995). What is sarcopenia? The Journals of Gerontology Series A: Biological Sciences and Medical Sciences, 50(Special Issue), 5-8.

Rolland, Y., Czerwinski, S., Abellan Van Kan, G., Morley, J. E., Cesari, M., Onder, G., ... & Vellas, B. (2007). Sarcopenia: Its assessment, etiology, pathogenesis, consequences and future perspectives. The Journal of Nutrition, Health & Aging, 11(6), 486-495.

Institute of Medicine. (2005). Dietary reference intakes for water, potassium, sodium, chloride, and sulfate. National Academies Press

Centers for Disease Control and Prevention. (2021). Falls among older adults: An overview. https://www.cdc.gov/falls/facts.html

Shelley Carrol MPT

www.ingramcontent.com/pod-product-compliance
Lightning Source LLC
Chambersburg PA
CBHW060518030426
42337CB00015B/1930